True Confessions of a Veterinarian

True Confessions of a Veterinarian:
AN UNCONDITIONAL LOVE STORY

Gene Witiak, V.M.D.

Glenbridge Publishing Ltd.

Illustrations

Patricia Hobbs

Copyright © 2004 by Gene Witiak

Published by Glenbridge Publishing Ltd.
19923 E. Long Ave.
Centennial, Colorado 80016

Library of Congress Catalog Card Number: LC 2003115314

International Standard Book Number: 0-944435-54-8

10   9   8   7   6   5   4   3   2

To

"Jemima"
She Never Stopped Giving

With special thanks to Dawn Lennon, editor/agent,
my dear family,
and to all of you who put your trust in me.

CONTENTS

Prologue   1

I. You Named Your Pet *What*?   5
II. Pearls   20
III. Just Another Day at the Office!   45
IV. "Doctor, Is It Serious?"   77
V. Children and Their Pets   101
VI. If It's Not One Thing, It's Another!   111
VII. Swallowed Objects   130
VIII. There is No Love in Calories!   142
IX. Tough Choices — Right Decisions   155
X. The Home Front   166

Epilogue   196
A Final Tribute   206

PROLOGUE

True Confessions

Before you get too far here, there are some things you need to know about me. Some may surprise you, some may touch you, some may irk you, and some may just make you laugh — yes, at me. I have been a veterinarian for over forty years, so I have met a lot of people and a lot of pets. Some have made me laugh too — and cry and fume and beam with joy. I've written here about memorable moments, relationships, and discoveries from my shared experiences with people and their pets. Their stories have become my story, so I need to own up to some truths before we begin.

CONFESSION #1:   As a kid I never had a pet. In college I'd planned to become a dentist. But once I realized that people sitting in a dentist chair, mouths filled with instruments, couldn't talk with me, I decided to become a veterinarian. At least even if my patients couldn't say anything, their owners could. Human connection is important to me.

CONFESSION #2:   I don't just *like* people, I enjoy them. I don't just *love* animals, I respect them. When I care for a pet, I help a family and that makes me happy.

CONFESSION #3:   I can be a wise guy. Human foibles (my own included) and peculiar circumstances that involve people and their pets make me laugh. I use them to try to make others laugh because sometimes that's the only relief available. Life isn't always easy in a veterinary practice.

CONFESSION #4:   Labrador retrievers are my favorite breed — they have been our family canine companions for over forty years. All right, I personally relate to Labs in many ways: they are funny, loving, and seemingly optimistic about nearly everything. I'm like that too, only I think I'm a bit smarter. You can be the judge of that.

CONFESSION #5:   I am Christian by birth and a member of the Episcopal church by choice — so I know a fair number of members of the cloth and am inclined to see liturgical connections in my life experiences. Hopefully, you'll forgive me for that. Please know, however, that I hold in high regard all approaches to spiritual celebration — love has no bounds. Anyone with a pet knows that too, that's for sure.

CONFESSION #6:   Confessions 4 and 5 have formed the basis of my fantasy job — to be the Vatican's veterinarian.

In that unique capacity I would be positioned to convince the powers-that-be to designate the Labrador retriever as the official dog of the Vatican. My strategy and studied arguments are presented in the Epilogue where you too are invited to weigh the evidence.

CONFESSION #7: After forty years as a veterinarian, I see a lot of things in life more clearly now, particularly the lasting relationships that can grow between a veterinarian and his/her clients and patients. I have had some of the same clients for decades, following the lifetimes of a string of their pets.

On the basis of these true confessions, I offer you this veterinarian's love story — a series of tales about the people and the pets that I have known and cherished. They have made me laugh and cry, but more importantly, they have made me better. Because of my life experiences and this profession, I have come to know that there are no greater feelings than being loved, wanted, and needed.

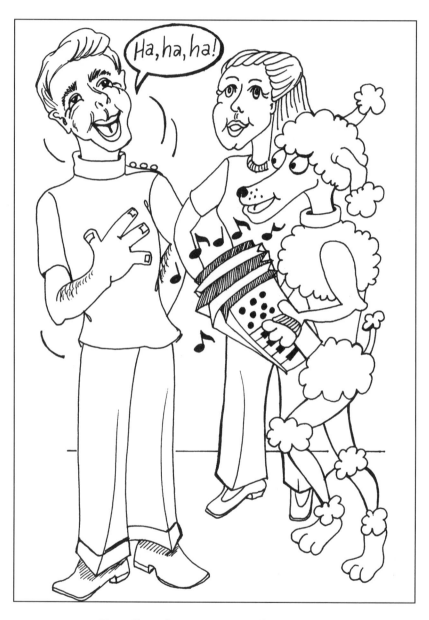

Peculiar circumstances that involve
people and their pets make me laugh.

CHAPTER I

You Named Your Pet *What?*

The first words we utter to our precious new pets always seem to be, "Now, what am I going to call you?" From this our unconditional love stories begin.

The question, "How did your pet's name come about," generally leads to interesting veterinary office conversation. The naming process can be a unique experience depending upon the family. There may be occasional controversy but total family involvement can be very important.

Some families let each member submit a name, and then all the choices are voted on democratically. I love that. The reasons given for pet names are many and the thought processes often pretty unique.

We're all familiar with books that prospective parents use as a resource to select their children's names. One year "Emily" and "Matthew" outdistance all other names, and another year the premier name may be "Alison" or "Michael." Pet names, on the other hand, tend not to come from a book — they come from, well, us!

"Oh, she just looks like a 'Fluffy.' "

"He reminded me of an old friend."

"Well, she was born near Christmas."

"She's so black, what would *you* have named her?"

"He's just like our last one."

"Sure, we found him along a highway."

One day I asked Mrs. Freedman why she named her cat "R.C." "Well, she's a heckuva mouser, so R.C. is 'rodent control' for short."

"Jim, 'Mohammed' is an interesting name for your collie pup. Give me some background."

"Well, Doc, I'm a huge boxing fan, so he became 'Mohammed Collie (call-ee).' " Ten years earlier his name probably would have been "Cassius Collie."

"From your description of the kitten's escapade, I daresay your name selection is apropos," was my response to Dorothy's naming story.

The police arrived on the scene following her "emergency" call — no, this was not the 911 variety but clearly a situation that needed professional help. A homeless kitten was caught by its neck in a chain-link fence. This was a very frightened, stray feline.

Soon that familiar blue can of hydrogenated fat made its appearance. A welcomed application of this baker's goo made this two-pound kitty as slippery as an eel and freed it from its entrapment. So it made perfect sense to call him the "Crisco Kit."

A new client came in with a recently adopted kitten for a wellness exam. A complete history was obtained revealing that the owner was an educator, born and raised locally, and that, a generation ago, I had treated her parents' pets. And, oh yes, her kitten was doing well and had been wholeheartedly endorsed by her two adult feline housemates. Well, a complete history is a *complete* history.

She had named the kitten "T.C." (Remember R.C. previously?) T.C. wasn't "The Cat" as I had supposed, but rather "Treble Clef." And why not? She was joining a cat family that included "Jazzy" and "Notez." No, this "sharp" client wasn't a music teacher but rather a music-loving librarian.

"With a yellow Lab named 'Trauma,' I assume that you're affiliated with the medical field in some way," I said to this new client.

"Yes, I'm a paramedic with our township's volunteer ambulance service," replied this attractive young mother.

I then went on to tell her, "As unusual as your dog's name is, she's the second Trauma that I see regularly. The other is also a

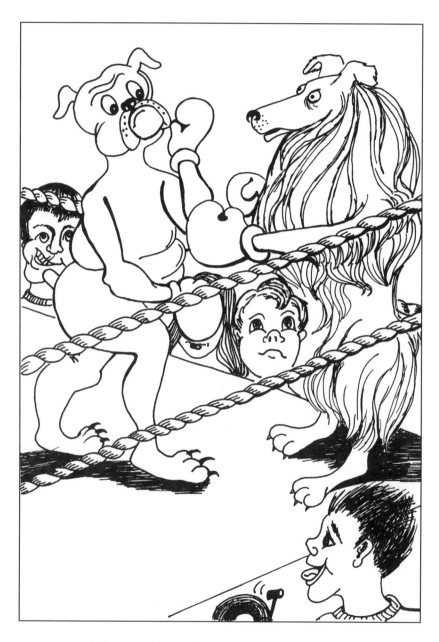

His name is Mohammed Collie (call-ee)

blonde, but a cocker spaniel. Her owner, Bill, is an emergency medical technician in a neighboring township as well."

"That's not Bill Lester, is it?"

Well, yes, it was and she had known him professionally for years but had never compared canine notes with him. Fortunately, no one was left *traumatized* by this situation.

"Doctor W., you told me you'd never forget my cat's name," the librarian said to my wife, Joan, and me as we were checking out a few books at our local library. I couldn't recall the woman's name, let alone her pet's name, a feline I had seen perhaps eight to ten months earlier.

I stammered for a few moments and said, "It's 'Nicodemus.'" She looked at me in a startled fashion, and I knew my guess was incorrect. "Nope, but a least you got the right book. It's 'Deuteronomy.'"

Not long thereafter, Deuteronomy's owner died. I went to the viewing and was amazed at the huge throng of people there to offer their sympathies to her family and to honor this dear lady who loved her cats. Deuteronomy still comes in with his dad now, and I promised myself never again to forget that dear cat's name.

Over the years, names regularly have eluded me. When I bump into a client while I'm out shopping, I'm darn good at saying, "Oh, yes, you have the black dachshund who wets the floor when I pick him up." I think people like their veterinarians to remember their pets even to the exclusion of themselves. If I meet a client and don't remember his name or the pet's, I'm quick to say, "How unusual it is for me to see you without your sweet poodle." Or "How is the lady whose cat likes our office about as well as I like the dentist's chair?"

In my family, we've always favored "people names" for our cats and dogs. A few of ours include "Annie, Dinah, Ernie, Sara, Bonnie, Ben, Moses, Jemima, Sophie, Simon, Dawn, Rosie, Elizabeth, Walter, Jacob, and Lu-si." Lest you think our home is overrun with pets, realize that most of these loved ones have passed on.

"Annie" is our Burmese cat that I had flown in as a surprise for my wife on our twenty-fifth anniversary, hence the name "Annie-versary." Joan panicked for a few short seconds as she looked into the carrier at her gift since the chocolate-colored kitten looked like a ferret! Her momentary shock became instantaneous love.

We decided to keep Annie in our bedroom for several days to acclimate her to her new surroundings and to spare her from the overwhelming attention expected from our two Labs and one other cat. She immediately adopted a sleeping position under the covers in the warmth of my wife's partially flexed knees. As a result, she quickly acquired the nickname of "B.C.," short for birth control. Her adjustment period was over quickly as the pet population in our household just had to know what was going on in the bedroom.

People occasionally will go to pick out a kitten and then not be able to leave that "last one" behind. So I often get to see twins at that first office visit. I have a feeling that litter owners, in this situation, bring out another "last" kitten in hopes that softheartedness will result in a new home for two.

All veterinarians see these littermates with names such as "Amos and Andy, Fred and Ethel, Puss and Boots, Mutt and Jeff, Anthony and Cleopatra, Bartles and James, Cagney and Lacey, Jack and Jill, Ike and Mike" and on and on.

Canines of unknown lineage used to be termed mongrels — how demeaning! Over time, the term "mixed breed" was preferred. And now, being more sensitive to actual lineage, I've come to use kinder and more accurate terms like Lab/setter cross.

When a cuddly creature of questionable background, but with redeeming features and great character, is presented to me for examination, I am inspired to bestow genuine respect for their lineage: "This pet, henceforth, shall be called a 'Hollywood shag dog.'" "Mandy" was part of our practice for fourteen years, and this breed designation befitted her. New members of our staff would say they had never heard of a Hollywood shag dog (HSD, for short). Veteran staff members then feigned genuine shock over their apparent "ignorance."

Annually, we were invited to a Christmas cocktail party at a dear friend's house. During a lull in the conversation, I could hear our hostess telling a guest with the greatest of pride, "Why, she's a Hollywood shag dog — very popular on the West Coast, but relatively new to the area. Aren't many around here." That made me feel quite proud. I'll never ever see a purebred Hollywood shag dog, but who knows, maybe a Lab/HSD cross one day.

A beautiful foundling came to our practice two years back with a very questionable heritage. This streamlined, six-month-old creature looked both athletic and graceful. My keen sense of breed determination led me quickly to pronounce him a Kenyan antelope hound. With a look of both amusement and dismay, his owner stated that a friend of hers had that feeling also — that the dog reminded her of Africa.

The following week I received this typewritten letter:

Dear Gene,

After much research I find you are mistaken about the country of origin of my dog, "Freddy." He is not a Kenyan antelope hound but an *Egyptian* antelope hound.

This breed was known as far back as the Egyptian Middle Kingdom 2040-1783 B.C. The dog-headed God of the Dead (Anubis) was probably modeled on this breed. As one can see from the enclosed illustration, the resemblance is striking.

Anubis was worshipped not only in Egypt but also in Greece. The center of this cult was in the city of Kynopolis, which as you know, means "dog city" in Greek.

He was still worshipped in Rome circa 100 A.D. Apuleius describes him as "rearing terrifically high his dog's head and neck. . .alternately a face black as night and golden as the day." It is not known when the antelope hound was brought to Kenya where you saw them, but the breed became popular for game hunting when the British took over the country in the 1880s.

Hemingway acquired a pair of these dogs while he was writing *The Green Hills of Africa.* (Unfortunately, his

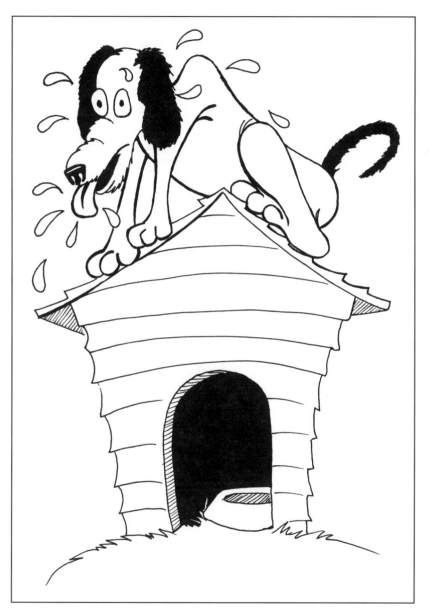

My grandfather climbed
Mt. Kilimanjaro, and I can barely get up here.

dogs were cropped out of the photo I sent you.) It is claimed that they climbed Mt. Kilimanjaro with him but I feel this is a canard. While their lung capacity is great, I doubt they could climb to 19,340 feet.

My dog is much admired for his looks and gentle nature. People who meet him wonder why there are not more of these hounds in America.

I would appreciate it very much if you would correct your records to show the correct nomenclature for this breed.

My best to you and Joan,

I had met my match and then some! Quite a payback, and deservedly so, from a brilliant woman of many fine words. Such are the perils of my naming "genius"!

Many years ago, on a memorable Monday night, a middle-aged, medium-sized canine was brought to me by its new owner. "Doc, it's a mixed breed I picked up just last week."

I decided then and there that this alert-looking, setter-sized adoptee with tail a-wagging deserved better than our "mixed breed" designation on his medical record. Immediately, I selected the breed to be a "Roanoke setter." Stunned, Mr. Owner said, "Guess where I returned from this weekend? My job took me to Roanoke, Virginia, last Monday." Lucky guess? Who knew?

A rottweiler-boxer mismating resulted in a pup that came to the office with its handsome owner, so I immediately informed him of my penchant for developing new breeds. As a result, this youthful male pup became the original "boxweiler" in the canine kingdom. Not five minutes later from the waiting room, I heard his owner declare that a more accurate breed label was needed to reflect his uniquely Germanic stature and would be more appropriate. Hence, I dubbed him the "Lithuanian boxweiler," and before me stood the crown prince of this "new" breed.

The above happened on a Thursday and the following Monday, the significance of the event truly unfolded. A mother and her college-age son were in for an office visit with their seventeen-year-old cat, a patient we had never seen. She had the typical ammoniacal odor of renal failure, and thirty minutes later the blood chemistries corroborated the diagnosis. This family had decided to have her euthanized because of her failing health, damaged kidneys, and her age. This decision was both kind and proper.

While waiting for the results of the blood tests, our conversation turned to the origin of their family last name. "What background is Daxx?" I inquired.

"Why, my husband's grandparents are from Lithuania." Well, you might well guess how quickly the previous Thursday's events tumbled into our conversation about the Lithuanian boxweiler. There is no question in my mind that these two events occurred as if by divine intervention, as they, to a small degree, eased the sadness of the pending euthanasia, or at the very least, were a distraction.

I'll often ask clients, "Where did you get your new pet?" Sometimes the client will shyly explain that it came from the humane society or a pet store, offering the information as something of an apology. In my view, these are very lucky pets that probably had little or no love in their prior homes and now have found a family where they will be safe and loved. No one should ever think the origin of their pets is important — it is the pet itself that matters and the relationship that will grow between it and its human family.

A pet bought from a home environment goes from a home full of love to another loving household. I sometimes think the pets that come from "sad" places appreciate their new loving homes a lot more.

A feral cat came into our family's life in November 1997. We had seen him over the summer months in the woods behind our house. He staggered as he walked, showing little coordination, was badly matted and, expectedly, was extremely shy.

·   It took about two weeks to snare him in a borrowed Humane Society trap. This Have-a-Heart trap was a lifesaver for this feline of very suspect origins. Our intention was either to euthanize him if he was unmanageable or to neuter, vaccinate for rabies, and then release him. I was alone in an exam room as I donned our up-to-the-elbow cowhide gloves, opened the crate, and waited for the "attack cat" to exit.

"Mr. No Name," at this point, crept out of the trap using his olfactory sense and, in a flash, was diving into a plastic container of dog treats on top of the counter. After de-gloving, I reached a gentle hand to acclimate him to my presence. Within moments he was in my arms, a skinny, heavily-matted, purring machine. A quick exam revealed he was already neutered. We named him "Moses."

Obviously, he had been a drop off with a never-to-be-determined affliction of his central nervous system that occurred either from birth or from some head trauma. To this day he has to lean against the back or side walls of our house to urinate or defecate in our flower beds.

Moses is spending another winter with us now. His heated, pillowed, and insulated box graces our garage. Our two Labs and he have become like the Three Amigos. He stumbles after them and lies in the sun with them. One of the dogs licks him constantly, and the mutual acceptance is truly remarkable. Yearly, I take him to the office and comb out his mats; a few are clipped out. He purrs, as daily he is picked up, and lies like a baby in your arms. He even enjoys the plucking of his entwined hairs.

Although he didn't have to part the Red Sea, this Moses truly found the Promised Land, unquestionably giving as much as he received. I cannot imagine how he survived in the sixteen acres of woods behind us, being unable to catch anything to eat. How sad it is even to imagine that life. Our family was blessed when he found us.

The origin of the pet names is an endless source of amazement to me. Here's how some of these conversations go:

"It's like this. We found this cat in a church parking lot and it seemed a logical choice. We took him to our neighborhood veterinarian before we moved here. In all honesty, we had named him 'Nun,' but after his exam, he was renamed 'Monk.' "

" 'Barre' for a feline name is unusual. How did this come about?" I asked.

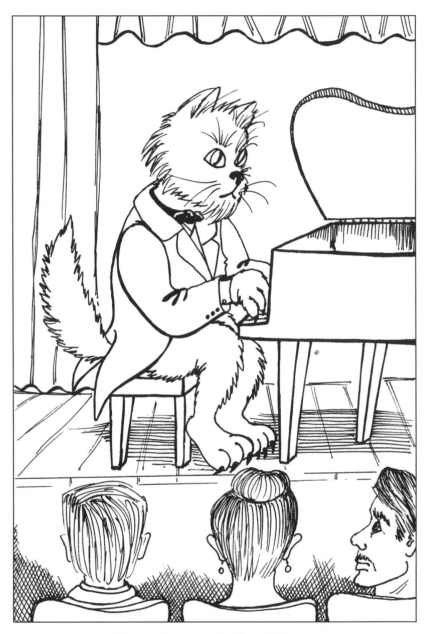

The cat's name is Van Cliburn.

"We plucked him from the median strip of a four lane highway near Wilkes-Barre, Pennsylvania."

"So, did you name her 'Dumpling' because she was a wide-bodied kitten?" I queried.
"Nope, found her in a dumpster."

Each special name begins a lifelong connection that grows strong through shared experience and love. This unconditional love between owner and pet says, "I'll always be there for you."

CHAPTER 11

Pearls

Pearls come from sea creatures and are truly gems. Whether worn as a strand or alone, they are beautiful to behold. Pearls are like old friends, and over the years many of my clients have become my pearls. These clients are gems both to my practice and to me.

This chapter is named for one of my all-time most memorable clients — a very special lady named Pearl.

She and her husband, Tony, came to our practice about twenty-five years ago with a Gordon setter named "Maggie" who had developed urinary incontinence secondary to a lack of estrogen. About one half of one percent of female dogs that are spayed (ovariohysterectomized) develop this syndrome. Today this problem is usually responsive to the antihistamine phenylpropanolamine (PPA), but in those days veterinarians only had diethylstilbestrol (estrogen) as a treatment. Even now, in a small percentage of cases, we resort to the old hormone.

For a Gordon setter, the dose was 1 pill daily for 5 days and then 1 pill twice a week thereafter. This was the dose I prescribed for Maggie. Two weeks after her visit, Pearl said to me over the phone: "Doc, Maggie's in heat, and as you know, she'd been spayed years ago." I jokingly replied that she had misread my directions on the pill envelope and had mistakenly given her the pills twice *daily* instead of twice *weekly*. At that level, the drug would produce breakthrough vaginal bleeding, simulating a heat cycle in the spayed female.

Within the hour Pearl was at the office taping onto my wall-mounted veterinary diploma her pill envelope with the directions stipulating "1 pill twice daily." Yes, it was in my handwriting! That tape turned yellow before the envelope finally disappeared from our office several years later.

My own Labs have become veggie lovers because of Pearl. She is a remarkably successful "small farmer," raising seeds to plants every spring for her friends, including me. My own successful garden, though only about 300 square feet, is also a tribute to Pearl. Tomatoes, peppers, broccoli, parsley, and the eighty lettuce plants (six varieties) that she delivered early every spring, resulted in a great vegetable crop that contributed to fifty consecutive nights of salad.

Each of our Labs over the years has carried a large brown shopping bag in her mouth during lettuce picking. When the salad spinner comes out in the kitchen and the bag rests comfortably on the floor (with some saliva on it, of course), the dogs sit at attention. They know that with the breaking of the lettuce, they will be rewarded with the hearts of that leafy vegetable. That's *one* healthy treat. You mean your dog doesn't have salad with its dinner!

Recently, Pearl's Doberman was due for a semiannual thyroid function test. This breed, like the golden retriever, is very prone to hypothyroidism (underactive function of the thyroid gland). In general Dobies and golden retrievers look at food and gain weight and often have a dull, sparse coat. The blood test for this condition is run on a serum sample four to six hours after receiving medication at home.

I personally dialed Pearl's number to tell her that we had a cancellation and she could come in later that morning. She gave a typical comment, "Well, I'm not dressed yet." I told her that any garb was suitable for a trip to our office and to take her time as we were in no hurry.

About fifteen minutes after her expected arrival time, the phone rang. Julie (Pearl's *other* best friend at our office) answered; the pallor in her face and shaky voice belied her anxiety. A police officer was describing a vehicle that had skidded across a roadway and was upside down with a woman trapped in the driver's seat, saved only by her seat belt. The woman's second statement to the officer was that she was going to be late for 'Katie's" blood test and could he possibly call us. Her first concern was that her dog had taken off in fright following the accident. The irony here was that she worried about everyone else before she thought of herself. That's not at all surprising if you knew this kind, faithful woman as well as I do.

We have clients who don't show up for appointments and those who come late, fouling our schedules and never offering an apology. Those who do apologize I hold in the highest regard. Goodness knows I've been late too for church, tennis, golf, and the list goes on and on — and then there's Pearl.

It took us about forty-five minutes to close up the office and reach the accident scene. The demolished car was settled on the flatbed, the fire police were rerouting traffic, and the ambulance was already hospital-bound with our gem of a friend.

Along with others, we walked the woods and rural neighborhoods unsuccessfully searching for Katie. Several hours later she turned up on the back porch of someone who recognized her. She had crossed a major highway and by some sixth canine sense, selected an appropriate recovery site.

A call to our local hospital revealed that, indeed, Pearl had been admitted through their emergency room. That night I visited with her for about an hour and she never let go of my hand. She was in excruciating pain every time she made the slightest movement. I could sense it in her face and through our hand contact. She did admit to discomfort but, true to form, did not want to upset me or seek my sympathy.

Pearl offered two possible causes for her accident, mechanical or physiological, meaning the car or her. Mechanical always implies a malfunctioning automobile. How often we hear senior citizens blame their accident on the mechanical failure of their car. Surprising no one, Pearl put the onus on herself. She frankly said that she didn't remember much of what had occurred.

At the hospital it was determined that she had a concussion, pinched cervical spinal nerves, and two fractured vertebrae. The prospects of an eighteen-day hospital stay did not sit well with this overactive bundle of gardening delight, now in her seventy-seventh year. After all, she was a very busy woman with no time to be off her feet!

To this day, though, she is in constant pain alleviated only somewhat by medication.

From that time on, she would be driven to our practice or we would go to her. When Pearl and her pets need us, we are there for them.

In our practice, we so appreciate client referrals that we award a gift certificate to anyone who sends us a new client. Accompanying the certificate is always a personal, hand-written note of thanks from me. I would like to claim that these notes are always hand-written solely for the reason of personalizing them. In truth, my typing ranks up there with my ability to knit and tap dance. I have never taken a typing course throughout my career and keep my distance from a computer. Conveniently, my wife is a computer/internet devotee. (Sadly, she has failed in her attempts to teach me to play solitaire on that mysterious piece of office equipment.)

I will never forget the O.R. nurse from a local hospital coming in with her referral gift certificate. Neither she nor I could decipher my handwriting well enough to determine just whom she had referred and was being thanked for. But she allowed that it was this personal touch that truly mattered.

I first met this nurse as a favor to a plastic surgeon for whom she worked. At the time, the veterinarian she used would not castrate her pet rat. I accepted the challenge readily.

Each of us had expectations that were clouded that morning. She was greeted by our veterinary assistant and asked to fill out the new client form. Her pet, "Sebastian," was no where to be seen. I walked to the counter to introduce myself to this attractive, bespectacled, and long-haired, young lady. After the usual discussion about mutual friends at St. Luke's Hospital (for people), my curiosity could wait no longer. "Did you decide against the surgery this morning?"

She pulled back her lengthy tresses and there sat Sebastian wrapped around her neck with his tail acting the part of a short necklace.

Sebastian's owner had used him for breeding purposes over the years, and many of his offspring graced research labs. As he reached his later years, I think he was grateful I had ended his tiring, breeding career. He was the best — and only — pet rat I've ever handled to this day. He never held his subsequent surgical procedure against me, as I handled him several times annually to trim his nails and shorten his teeth.

Over the years, my arrival home each evening would prompt a discussion about "my day at the office" from an inquisitive, caring wife. "I saw my favorite client of all time today," I'd answer.

"Then she's tied for first place, because nine out of the last ten nights you had your favorite in for a visit," she'd reply.

We would discuss not only which of our personal friends came to the office that day but also any and all interesting cases. This was a good cathartic time for each of us as she parented our twin daughters for the twelve hours a day that I was away at the practice.

"He didn't give me my pills," I overheard the octogenarian telling our receptionist after his office visit. I walked into the waiting room, reached across the counter, and deftly plucked the pill envelope from Sherwood's shirt pocket. (Seniors generally refuse childproof containers.)

A smile crept across his handsome face, and he asked if he could tell us a joke. We were happy to be his audience.

"Well now, it seems this elderly couple was watching television, and the husband says to the wife, 'Would you like some ice cream?' 'Sure,' she said. 'I'll have vanilla.' Several minutes later he returned with two fried eggs, and she asked, 'Where's my toast?'"

As is often the case, it's who tells the story and the circumstances at the time rather than the content of the tale. But that's always been Sherwood. He's a smiling, kind, trusting gentleman whose presence I always enjoy, not only because he could make you laugh but also because he could laugh at himself.

Every time he came in with one of his dogs, starting with "Scruffy" the poodle and then "Timmy" the beagle in the mid-'70s, he was spiffily attired. He would more often than not be clean-shaven, wearing a jacket and tie. Now the plaid jacket would sometimes clash with the checkered slacks and the striped shirt, but the hunting dog tie was always neatly in place.

But, you know what? Sherwood's genuine personality and kindly voice were all that mattered. Anyone would want him for a dad, including me. He is what is best described as huggable. But behind those smiling eyes was something profound. He was seeing a lady friend over in New Jersey and always had "to look his best." I never met her but she's a lucky woman.

Sherwood recently told me that his lady doesn't recognize him anymore, but that doesn't matter to this widowed gentleman; he still visits her.

Last year, I wrote a sympathy note to Sherwood on the loss of old "Sparky." Sparky was sixteen years old and had first been referred out for disc surgery. Most recently, he'd had his cancer-ridden spleen removed. Sparky's record showed up on my desk early one Monday morning. The sympathy note I sent to

Sherwood was on his loss, and, selfishly, for me also. Knowing that Sparky was gone meant that perhaps I'd never see Sherwood again.

Two months later, I heard Sherwood's voice in our waiting room, telling the receptionist that my note was much appreciated. But apparently, it may have been just a little premature, as there stood Sparky, straining at the end of his leash.

As I walked out to say "Hello," he said, "Doc, I know you're very efficient, but your kind note wasn't necessary quite yet!"

The Sparky that should have received the note had died at a local emergency center and someone had confused the last name. But as Sherwood later pointed out, "Two notes are better than none." Very recently, euthanasia did end Sparky's term on earth. Hugging this wonderful man at that sorrowful moment will always be remembered.

Sherwood called me several months after that about his granddaughter's Doberman pinscher who had a swollen ankle; he wanted me to look at it. It was an off weekend for me, but since I was to be at our hospital that Sunday planting more than a dozen shrubs and assuming they didn't mind my very nonprofessional attire, seeing "Ty" would be no problem. The fact that the Dobie was as nice as a Lab and his granddaughter was a personable young lady made the decision easy.

This note came in the mail a few days later. He's really a "pearl."

Dear Good Friend,

I want to thank you for taking care of Ty on Sunday. I came back to help you plant your shrubs but you were finished and gone.

Your friend,
Sherwood

Dorothy was born in 1907. (She wouldn't care that I gave out her birth year.) I tell you this for a good reason: she brought in a new schnauzer pup (a 10-month-old) in 2000.

She and I have "shared" five schnauzers in over thirty-two years of our relationship — two of them were diabetics. Her husband died in 1987, and to this day she lives alone in the house they built in 1941.

Dorothy retired from teaching in 1969. On more than one occasion I would introduce her to someone in the waiting room, and they would say, "I had you in junior high for Spanish or Latin, and you were the best teacher I ever had."

After many episodes of care for her dogs, I received a note typical of Dorothy's kind heart and feisty manner. Here is the core of it: "Dr. Witiak, I am writing this note to thank you for all your extra kindnesses — your phone calls, your visits to my home, and your caring for animals and people, especially for 'old ladies' like me. Someday, I'm really going to whack you with my cane!"

Six years ago her second diabetic dog, "Snoopy II," was euthanized. Dorothy was a single pet parent then and was eighty-seven years old, so what were the chances realistically of another pet for her? "Pinocchio" entered her life later that same year. He was an extremely well-bred schnauzer who, at his retirement from the show ring, was three years old. Although she paid an outlandish price for him, his gentlemanly personality made him well worth the cost.

At the age of nine, Pinocchio developed lymphoma and within two months died on Thanksgiving morning 2000. So now, enter "Pinocchio II." And although I would have claimed that his predecessor would be impossible to surpass, my first twenty minutes with this youngster led me to believe that he will have the same beautiful nature as number I. Realistically, Dorothy won't be here for his later years, but I'm 100 percent sure that her will includes a schnauzer trust fund.

Any chronicle about schnauzers would be incomplete without "Max, Chessie, TJ, Freida, Tara, Flicka I and II, and Alexa."

Surprisingly, none of these pets was ever named "Nittany" because this mature, but relatively newlywed couple, are serious college football fans of Penn State University. The 2000 season was disappointing for the football team in what would have been dubbed "Unhappy Valley," Pennsylvania. So this would be the first time in recent memory that this couple would be home on New Year's Day with their two schnauzers instead of at a bowl game. Oh well, togetherness at the start of a new year isn't all that bad.

One of my first memories in our friendship was in the early '70s. "Alexa," their two-year-old schnauzer, was hit by a car that resulted in a neck injury. Cervical spinal cord impingement produced a left front leg paralysis that ultimately led to amputation.

Between the time of the accident and the final result, this innovative couple did all in their power to avoid loss of that limb. Because Alexa was a healthy, robust youngster, they were driven to help her.

Alexa would drag the paralyzed leg, causing the top of the paw quickly to become ulcerated. Since Alexa had lost her pain receptors in that leg, she acted normally while unwittingly and unknowingly damaging her extremity. This was painful for the family to see.

To counter this, Martin went to a shoemaker who helped him devise a laceable leather boot. For a time this worked, but ultimately the pressure of the leather caused some tissue breakdown.

Our last effort was a consultation at our local community hospital. Jan, a neurosurgeon, and George, an orthopedic surgeon, committed themselves to a few gratis hours one afternoon. The three of us performed surgery to ankylose her carpus (wrist). Through the insertion of pins, permanent immobilization — known as ankylosis — is accomplished. It was reasonable to assume that the stiffened foot could now be placed on the ground, pad side down (the proper or ventral surface).

For a time there was some reason for optimism. But short-term success was quickly followed by failure. Although the wrist remained ankylosed, the body inherently rotated the leg at the elbow causing the foot to be dragged again upside down.

The success, if any, was that the owners, Chris and Martin, did everything possible for Alexa. My fondness for them all these years has only grown, and they have become very special to me. Their slightly compromised three-legged pet was as normal as the next one and every bit as loved for the rest of its life.

I remember a humorous story that a client told me about an extremely devoted owner who walked his elderly dachshund every morning, rain or shine. This was duly noted by Father Patrick of Holy Infancy Church, around whose parish property the pair had ambled for years.

One Sunday morning the priest noted the lonely man walking without his dog. "My son, I've watched over the years and have sensed the love you shared with your dog."

"Thank you, Father. Fritz passed on last evening," the man answered. "In fact, I was stopping by to see if I might bury him in the tree line at the back of your property."

"As much as I would like to grant you permission, the bishop has blessed this site, and it's considered hallowed soil and is most sacred," the priest replied.

"I had fully intended to donate $5,000 to your church building fund in Fritz's memory," the man responded.

"Why didn't you say Fritz was Catholic?" Father Patrick declared.

When a story begins, "A minister and a priest were. . ." I automatically wait for the punch line. In this next case, not so.

Gary is a Windish Lutheran minister and is married to Betty, a beautiful person, who just happens to be a minister also. You'd want either of these dog lovers to be your own best friend.

"Mozart," their decade-plus German shepherd, is just as likeable. His attitude is: "Oh well, I'm just at the vet's office, and he's a good friend of Mom and Dad. They sure do talk a lot. Just give my joints a good check, bring me my treats, and we'll be on our way."

On a recent visit, Betty told me this story. It seems Gary was away until late in the evening, so she and Mozart were enjoying a relaxing time together while she was watching TV or reading. As it turned out, the downstairs TV wasn't working but the one in the upstairs bedroom was fine. However, this senior shepherd could not manage the steps without Gary's help. So this was to be Betty's evening shared downstairs with her precious canine companion.

When Gary returned quite late that night from his work caring for his flock, he found his wife in watchful sleep over her beloved Mozart in what I have now come to call the "House of the Three Shepherds."

The only client that I ever taught the proper method of anal gland emptying was an Episcopal priest named Peter. When Peter was without his collar, he dazzled those around him with his bow tie. I always questioned whether those ties were clip-ons, so he would untie and then retie them in my presence to prove his manual dexterity — an essential requirement for emptying those glands rectally. Anal glands are analogous to a skunk's scent glands.

Over the years Peter was kept in fine supply of unsterilized surgical latex gloves to perform his canine anal gland duties. The two most important points I stressed with him were 1) never watch what you were doing and 2) don't perform this procedure in your living room.

I would recheck "Widget" when she came for her routine office visits. As I expected, Peter would faithfully clean her anal glands the morning of her appointment, and he was almost as good at this job as he was at getting his pastoral messages across during his sermons.

One day a gentleman brought his Portuguese water dog to the office with an ear problem. His wife had been in a few weeks earlier for the pup's final set of first year vaccinations. After introductions, he gave me a very inquisitive look and said,

"You're much younger than I thought you'd be." I, of course, was quite pleased at this compliment and inquired as to his statement.

"Well, my wife said that Pastor Peter married your daughter." (His reference was to the very same Peter so adept at anal gland emptying.) The fact that Peter is only three years my junior, however, did make that marriage prospect quite unrealistic. I was quick to recall, though, the most senior Senator Strom Thurmond and his young bride.

My curiosity had to be satisfied so I pursued the conversation further. "Your wife told you that my daughter was married to Pastor Peter? What!"

Putting two and two together, as veterinarians do daily, I figured out what had occurred. Besides being an Episcopal priest, Peter was headmaster of a local boarding school. The client's son attended that school where we had a mutual friend in Peter. Since Peter had performed the Sacrament of Matrimony at my daughter's wedding, I must have shortened my statement, saying "He married my daughter," while speaking to his wife. Surely, I much prefer having Peter as my dear friend rather than as a son-in-law!

How often in my later years have I said to my wife, "Don't you wish we had met them twenty years ago?" That only happens rarely, but when you meet someone special, you can just feel that chemistry.

He isn't a saint but his name is James and his father is a minister. James's family moved into a house directly across the street from us. And we just knew there was a special bond there.

Though much younger in age than we, friendship came naturally. His pert and vivacious, redheaded wife and their daughter of six (already the epitome of her mom) had a magnetic spirit of warmth and energy.

James's down-home humor was broadened by his funny Oklahoma accent that came by way of Baton Rouge, Louisiana. From his first days "up north," he noted how nice it was to see animals in the woods with fur because where he came from, all he was used to seeing were creatures with scales and a slithering locomotion.

Their animal kingdom at the time was "Copper," an adult cat with veterinary experience. That's the kind way of saying she disliked Pennsylvania veterinarians about as much as the southern variety. Okie, Cajun, Yankee, no matter; she took no prisoners.

"Would she accept a kitten?" is a fairly commonly asked question of veterinarians. So when James asked it, I put the focus back on him. "Do *you* think Copper would accept one?"

An awkward moment follows this question all too frequently. When a present house pet rejects a new addition during the trial period, there is generally much upset in the household. The love that develops for the newcomer quickly equals the love felt for that "old friend." It's amazing how love develops whether it's during a twenty-minute trial or a ten-year stay. When the trial doesn't work out, it's never easy to return the newcomer because of that immediate attachment. That is especially true when children are involved.

James has always been an easy mark for his two female housemates who really wanted a kitten, particularly a loveable, holdable orphan. So he and I discussed the possibilities and decided it was time to give it a try. We would find a kitten and introduce it to Copper.

Like most veterinary practices, ours routinely receives calls, especially in springtime, about available litters of kittens: "Free to good home; housebroken." (These ads always make me chuckle because it takes about eight minutes to litter-train a feline.) So we put out feelers for James and family. Soon thereafter our neighbors picked up "Angel" from our office. It seems she had been waiting there just for this opportunity. Timing is everything.

With the introduction of "Angel," Copper's routine was upset but tolerance came quickly; however, acceptance was never fully achieved. Angel was only two years old when we received a 10:30 Saturday night phone call with apologies. (Certainly this was unnecessary with such good friends.) As it turns out, Joan and I had just returned from a wedding reception, and I was in the process of changing my clothes. Subsequently, I appeared at our neighbor's front door wearing a white shirt, tie, and tennis shorts — but my outfit went totally unnoticed.

Indeed, their young cat was in dire straits with obvious signs of renal failure. By 1 AM our heavily utilized emergency center had corroborated the presumptive diagnosis of kidney failure. The blood tests had values that denied life. Although supportive fluids were continued Sunday, the repeated tests — thirty-six hours later — were every bit as poor. For good and kindly reasons, euthanasia was provided for this beloved youngster. Fittingly, Angel is now helping raise beans and tomatoes in our garden. She is in good company with members of our own "animal family" who have passed on.

Dogs, like children (in most cases), welcome discipline, and it was delightful to witness the interaction between neighbor and dog. It is exciting to see the sense of accomplishment in any youngster whose love of animals becomes so apparent.

One day I was surprised to see Lauren in our side yard teaching our dogs to jump over a person lying prone on the ground — her mother! It was impossible to tell which of the participants was having more fun. Or was it the observer? Most assuredly the Labs, who were enthralled with the activity, eagerly awaited the "rewards" planned for them — that yummy Milk Bone or gourmet cookie that our neighbors always offered.

Later Lauren called to say that, after a family discussion, they thought it was time for a new kitten. So a trip was organized to our local humane society. The jaunt included not only Lauren, Dad, and their doctor (me!) but also Granny from Oklahoma.

For a parent, moments like this should be recorded. There is such joy in seeing a young lady pick out her most prized possession for the next decade and a half. Predictably, her phone calls from college will always start with "How's 'Belle' doing? Oh yes, and how's Dad?"

Most recently, Patti called to tell me about a conversation with her daughter, Lauren, who asked, "Mom, if I get all A's in school, will you and Dad allow me to volunteer at the Humane Society where we picked out Belle?" If that didn't give goose bumps to her parents and me, nothing would. You know the ending. She works as a humane society volunteer with her mom, helping to find loving homes for lonely pets.

Arlene was quite angry with me about a decade ago. She died recently and I felt this tale should be told. The property where we lived for nearly thirty years had a three-foot-wide strip of grass outside our split-rail fence. Unfortunately, it was also 300 feet long and tapered down to a four-lane highway with a speed limit of 55 mph.

I always faced traffic when mowing this strongly sloped lawn since cars and trucks would be whizzing by only a few feet away. Whenever a car beeped I gave the usual wave, "Sure, I recognize you." One day it seems that my acknowledgment was unnoticed as I sensed a car doing a U-turn near where I was mowing. The next thing I knew, a red compact was stopping lawnside, causing traffic to veer into the remaining space in the southbound lane.

"I thought you were mad at me when I didn't see you wave," Arlene bemoaned. For safety reasons, I shooed her on her way and gave her a huge hug the next time she came in with "Duffy."

The year before she died, Arlene sent me my favorite Christmas card of all time. On the front was a photograph of a Christmas tree, a Wheaten terrier, and a very, very large stuffed dog that could easily be mistaken for another Wheaten. The real terrier was all slicked up in seasonal garb, including a Santa hat.

Inside was the expected season's greetings and penned in was, "Love to all" along with, "P.S. I'm so embarrassed. My mother made me do it." The photo will always adorn our waiting room. Duffy was the finest Wheaten terrier I'd ever met.

"Thanks Arlene, and here's my wave to you up there."

"Fuffy" was also a Wheaten terrier who belonged to our closest friends. They called our home one Memorial Day to say their canine had wandered off their property but had been seen in the neighborhood. The heavily traveled roads in their immediate vicinity were cause for great concern.

The problem was that every time Fuffy was called she came toward them and then sprinted off. Ultimately, after several hours, she stopped playing games and responded to their pleas to come to them.

The unanswerable quandary was what to do when she returned. Does she become the prodigal canine and receive praise and thanksgiving? Or does she deserve a reprimand?

Receiving accolades might let her think it is acceptable to run off at will only because she will return to untold kindness. Were she to be scolded, her next venture away might be longer as she anticipates a negative reception upon return.

After all these years, I am still at a loss for the proper reaction in this situation when a dog hasn't been trained to respond to the "Come" command. Since few dog owners accomplish this feat, the question remains open with me.

Her name is "Robin" and she comes in no matter what the weather — sun or rain, wind or snow. Over the years I have been fortunate enough to share in her many pets, both cats and dogs. They were all of the rescued variety, some even being adopted for her mom, which added to the opportunities to see her.

We have shared several extremely difficult, "kind-decision times" whenever euthanasia became the most humane alternative. But she shares so much more than that.

Every Christmas season for more than fifteen years she finds time to bake cookies and goodies for our staff. Along with these caloric indiscretions is delivered a beautifully handmade, tasteful woodcraft, each and every one of which adorns our home. In fact last year's gift is in our front perennial garden — a ladybug crossing. What could be more perfect!

"Amos" was a wonderful Lab, living well into the double-digit years. His owner was a delightful charmer originally from Charlotte, North Carolina. When Marjorie would ask Amos, "Would you rather go to Duke or be a dead dog?" he'd roll over playing dead as a doornail. The owner's Chapel Hill, Tarheel, Carolina-blue smile always showed off her pride. Of course I'll never forget his final house call. It was a privilege to care for him throughout his life and in his last moments. I was deeply touched by the tender note I received from Marjorie. Her words reminded me once again why I chose to be a veterinarian: "Thank you for ministering with such sensitivity to his [Amos'] family. Never once was I made to feel that you were too busy to care for us."

Marjorie's prideful moments with Amos were in stark contrast to her not so prideful moment about two years later when she brought "Tippy" in for her annual exam. Now Tippy was a domestic shorthaired cat quite long in the tooth. As a matter of fact, she would like to sink that aforementioned tooth into my hand, came the warning from the mistress.

"Not to worry," I said to myself. After all I'm an old pro. So I swaggered toward the scale with said feline filling my left arm. As the right arm reached out to adjust the scale that seventeen-year-old domestic shorthaired cat took on the outward behavior of a two-year-old as she twisted free with gnashing teeth and extended claws. I deftly maneuvered out of harm's way. Well, not exactly. The familiar warm feeling of a urine sample running down my shirt, tie, and trousers was readily apparent to all present.

Because of the senior status of this pet, we did a urinalysis on the deposited specimen — at least the part we could salvage off the floor. So the situation was not a total loss.

An embarrassed Marjorie immediately insisted that she pay for the cleaning bill. Of course her kind offer was not accepted. The rest of the office visit went uneventfully. That means a quick stethoscope to the chest with a glove-clad technician providing restraint, and two quick vaccinations. Well, at least, we knew Tippy's heart was beating, and there was no sugar in her urine.

Two weeks later a package arrived with this note:

> Dear Dr. W.,
>
> I'm so embarrassed, I feel like a *DOG*. Please accept my apology for my outrageous behavior.
>
> Your friend,
> Tippy

Accompanying the unique card was a top quality veterinarian's tie — tiny boxer dogs on a navy-blue background. It's so tasteful that I even wear it to church.

My return note had the expected words of thanks for the gift and the offer of a free urinalysis the next time Tippy was willing!

Lori is a short, vivacious lady who has four equally charming daughters. She has also passed her excellent genes for pet caring to her offspring. I specifically recall two incidents that occurred over the many, many visits we shared over the years.

Nine years ago an extremely handsome springer spaniel pup was sitting on the exam table. " 'Links' is his name, and you're right, Jim named him." Jim was out enjoying his favorite pastime, playing golf.

The pup had been purchased from a psychiatrist who had included a fifty-two page notebook describing lineage, feeding, vaccination history, etc. I was quite impressed until I read his explicit directions on how our practice was to carry out the pup's care. Suggestions are always fine, but this breeder had gone too far. A quick phone call to the breeder resolved our differences. Lori's upbeat personality helped ease the moment — all for the love of that pup.

The other event involving this family took place at a wedding reception at a local country club. By way of background, Lori is not only a good sport but also a great sports fan. They have season tickets for all four of Philadelphia's major sports teams. And she knows many of the players personally. Now back to the reception.

The 18th green on the club's Old Course is a wonderful backdrop for wedding photos. During the photo session with the entire wedding party, who comes walking up to the green but a foursome that included Charles Barkley, the 6 foot 5 inch tall, 270-pound "Round Mound of Rebound" of the Philadelphia 76ers basketball team.

Now "Sir Charles" has a history of being a bad, bad boy. But let it be known, he is truly loved by Philly fans as the ultimate "blue collar" worker. If only those sports afficionados who disliked him for whatever reason could have heard his affable exchanges at the photo session, they might feel differently. His first reaction to being asked to pose with the newlyweds was, "You want *me* in your wedding picture."

After this unique photo op, the bride exclaimed, "I thought my husband was a big guy, but not compared to Charles."

When I heard the story and viewed pictures of this big man posing with the wedding party and out-sizing this attractive group, I laughed. But even Charles's size and equally large smile couldn't outshine the beauty of the bride.

Chuck is eighty-three in age only. This personable, sprightly gentleman lost his wife of many years to cancer. Teentz was an elegant lady, both outside and in. She was Chuck's best and inseparable friend for their whole married life. They were fixtures every Sunday in the church we attended together.

His phone call two months ago both surprised *and* shocked me. "I just adopted [the surprise] an eleven-year-old rottweiler [the shock], and I'd like for you to see her as soon as possible."

"How about in fifteen minutes?" I was tempted to say! We made an appointment for him as soon as we could.

Later that week, the new "Dynamic Duo" made their appearance. Other than a floor covered with happy rottie hair and a smiling senior citizen, the visit was as normal as any other. A truly happy-go-lucky attitude applied to each of them.

"I know I've set myself up for sadness in the not too distant future, but I *am* on the other side of the mountain myself, Doc. My home is no longer empty. I again have a wonderful companion," was Chuck's explanation.

Chuck is now working with an excellent personal dog trainer and veterinary technician. This will help prevent his left arm from getting stretched by this large and enthusiastic buttwagger. After all, she weighs only twenty pounds less than her

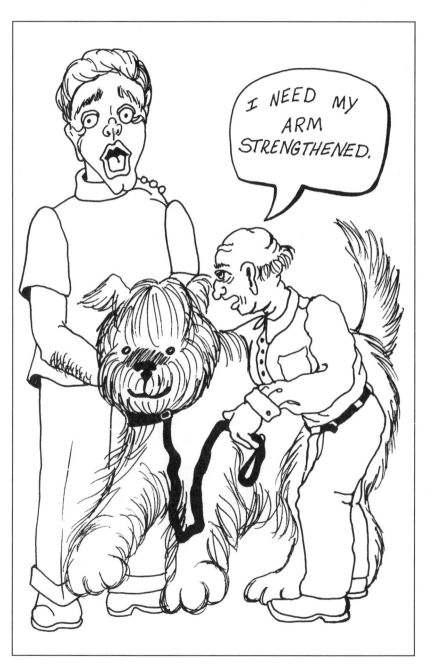

new owner who just saved her life and she, more than likely, lengthened his.

The joy of veterinary practice, as in life, comes from the relationships that grow from mutual caring. It's a beautiful thing when the love we have for our pets becomes a path to special human connection. In my world the relationship of client, pet, and veterinarian is unique and the rewards deep and lasting.

CHAPTER III

Just Another Day at the Office!

An office visit should encourage tolerance and, hopefully, acceptance by the pet. And if it takes fussing and hugging them to achieve that, all the better.

What better place to start a unique relationship among the owner, pet, and veterinarian than in the exam room. Through smiles, eye contact, and the right words, a climate of trust emerges. Empathetic listening and openness help to create a relaxed atmosphere that helps lessen the stress on all concerned, especially the pet. But it is no guarantee! How often a fractious dog comes into the exam room with that panicky attitude of "uh-oh, what's coming next!" In these circumstances, never ever think that nice guy tactics will always work. Far from it. You just can't risk misjudging the dog's reactions or trust the client's ability to interpret or manage its behavior. Surprise is usually the order of the day on both counts.

Sitting down with a client next to the dog to talk for a period of time will likely calm a developing situation. The owner relaxes as you discuss world matters, family, children, and, oh yes, the canine in front of you. The peace offering of a doggie treat (and when necessary a "Valium-impregnated" one!) is a good idea. Remember, it is important to know your audience as we will bear witness later.

Asking a cat to take a deep breath and hold it while placing a stethoscope against its chest is a must. An occasional owner questions this "tongue-in-cheek" requirement but, hopefully very rarely! Speaking loudly and directly into a geriatric dog's ear, often inspires conversation from their senior citizen owners.

On the exam table a new kitten's or pup's attitude is as variable as snowflakes. We'll sometimes see sleeping beauties and ask the owner, "Is our practice really that boring?" Or "could it be that the puppy is really here for an autopsy" (necropsy in veterinary terms) because it looks completely dead to the world and unresponsive. Then with the wave of a treat in front of those relaxed nostrils, we all share in the fun of seeing the young one arouse itself and begin "snacking."

Office visits aren't always this charming. A three-and-a-half pound schipperke pup recently came in with his elderly owner. It was his first visit to our practice. This little peanut of ten weeks would have bitten my cheek had he been able to reach it while his nails were being trimmed.

I noticed that the wrists of his gentleman owner looked rather bitten up, so I leaned over the table to unbutton his sleeves, surprising him. As expected, the skin was punctured just about up to the elbows.

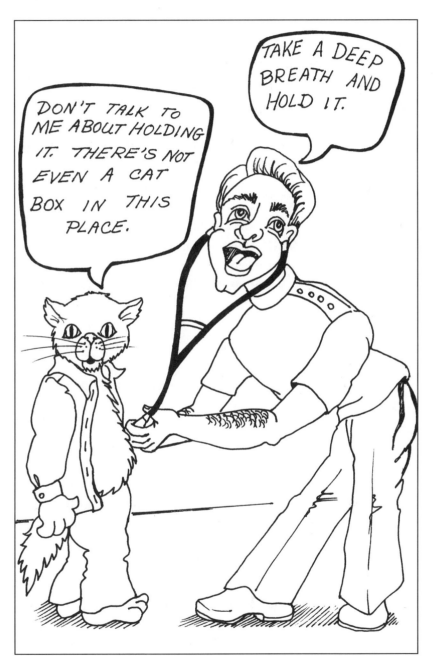

"Doc, my wife is an invalid, and she won't even let me scold the little guy."

"Well," I thought, "this 'little guy' will be fifteen pounds of fury for the next fifteen years of his life. Maybe I should consider retirement, or maybe I should be sick for their next trip to our office."

No employee of a veterinary practice ever forgets that group of pets kindly regarded as "caution." Their owners usually describe them in carefully chosen phrases that should put you on warning:

"He's a little shy with strangers."

"Walk up to him slowly and don't try to pet him."

"Let him come over to you."

"Let him sniff you and put the treat on the floor. Don't hand it to him."

"He's really good at home, only likes the family."

"Just doesn't like other dogs."

"I can handle him, Doc. He's just afraid of vets."

"His hackles are always up, doesn't mean a thing."

"She won't bite, wouldn't hurt a flea."

"The last vet muzzled him but we won't need one."

"Ever since the groomer cut her nails too short, she's foot shy."

And any staff member could add dozens more declarations to this list. Few owners will say that their pet is a nasty S.O.B that cannot be trusted. But you'd better believe those that do warn you!

As a veterinarian grows in experience, he or she also should be better able to evaluate the personality not only of the pet and its owner but also the relationship they share. Is the client credible in his statements? Can she truly handle the nine-pound Persian or the one-hundred-twenty-pound rottweiler?

A veterinarian must show ingenuity in his methods to keep in control of any and all situations without resorting to brute force. (Valium is always there as the great equalizer.) A superbly trained, well-schooled, trustworthy veterinary technician is the foundation for these times when support is needed. Often times, just knowing a tech is there and available allows the doctor to relax — something which, in itself, helps resolve many a challenge. I've hired and worked with many technicians over the years, and most have performed well beyond expectations. They've certainly saved me in more ways than one.

Case in point. "Rookie" was a mixed black retriever who was an extremely aggressive neutered male. Not one of our staff looked forward to the visit of this tennis ball-loving creature. Muzzling was out of the question as no staff member could get close enough.

Kelly, a seasoned technician and an excellent athlete, asked if I had the usual three or four cans of used tennis balls in my car. Before I knew it a few had been extracted from my trunk, one of which was quickly and proudly held in Rookie's mouth — a mouth, might I add, whose lips were drawn back in the infamous snarl position. He would not relinquish that ball come hell or high water. Needless to say, after that particular day, there was always a fuzzy yellow spheroid in our muzzle drawer, just in case Rookie forgot his own.

"Barney" was a different story. He was a gentle cairn terrier until it came time to perform a pedicure. His mom said that he was easily distracted at home no matter what, just by singing the "Barney song." I easily memorized the lyrics as they consisted of his name repeated over and over and over again with a slight pause after each third "Barney."

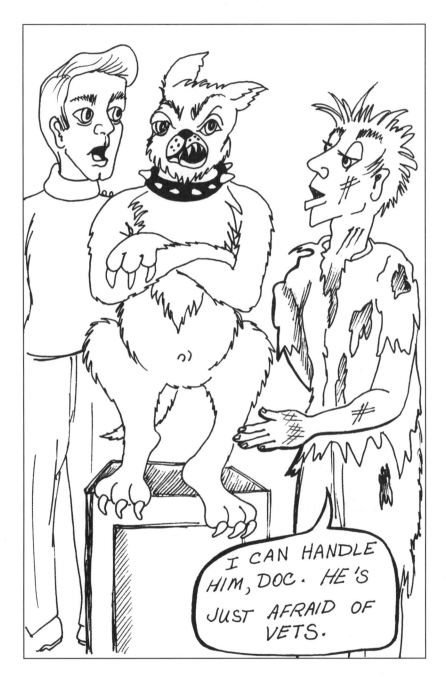

Over the years our Barney duet brought a lot of attention to that particular exam room. I was quite proud of this, never having made the first cut in church choir tryouts.

During a physical, of course, examination of teeth and gums is routine. However, this is limited to some degree by the nature of the beast. If the owner's complaint describes a sudden worsening of their pet's breath, and if this seems to correlate with a painful mouth, the nervous or shy pet probably requires sedation for a thorough mouth evaluation. Typical signs of oral cavity discomfort might be drooling, rubbing the lips, dropping food, or head tilting while chewing.

Pets, of course, can't talk or just maybe we don't listen. The signs of mouth problems are rather obvious. But an owner would never expect her pet to say, "Check my mouth, please." Your weekly mouth check should start at puppyhood. The earlier you discover a problem, the easier it is to resolve it.

Very recently, our thirteen-year-old Burmese cat was anesthetized for a dentistry. Our dental tech, Chris, suggested the extraction of the left, fourth upper premolar — a major tooth — because of bone loss allowing root exposure. Her experience and expertise made it a no-brainer. "Go for it," I concluded.

Seemingly the mouth never bothered "Bonnie," at least in our eyes. But eight weeks later, she acted more like a three-year-old rather than a decade-old cat, purring and "into things." She probably had a painful mouth but never told us. But just maybe we weren't listening.

Don't wait for head-shaking to examine the ears. Check them weekly and wipe out what you can see with handkerchief material moistened with otic solution, vinegar, or alcohol. Please practice pet prophylaxis.

"That sounds like preventive maintenance on my car," said a rather large jolly client. This was after we explained to him about the importance of checking his pup's teeth daily so as to get him used to it. We then added to the list one of my favorites: "Stick a finger in your dog's ear weekly. Then repeat the process with the other ear using a different finger. Then compare them using your eyes and your nose!"

If both ears are odor free and clean, repeat the process in seven days and then for, oh, about the next fifteen years! With any sign of an early problem, then clean the ear for three days straight. If there is no resolution, call your veterinarian.

This truly is preventive maintenance, oops! medicine, because you discover problems before your pet tells you about them. Both your car and your pet will be better for it.

I am of the (minority) opinion that dogs get headaches. Our practice is certain that "Arthur," the terrier, does and it is so indicated on the top of his hefty chart. This presumptive diagnosis is based on Arthur's having exceptionally clean, normal appearing ears despite head shaking and ear rubbing. He has no obvious allergies and has an excellent response to aspirin. By just listening to your dog, you too can nip a potential headache in the bud.

A great part of veterinary practice is education. Frequently I arrive home with an artistic reproduction penned onto my left hand. "Guess there wasn't any scrap paper available at work today" is the usual comment by one of our children.

What better way to demonstrate on the spot the size differences of ticks by sex. Or the difference between the common brown dog tick and the deer tick (the one that carries lyme disease). Or how to assess the reproductive tract of the female pet in varying stages of pregnancy. I did more of this before the invention of the indelible felt-tip pen — permanent diagrams on my person were never part of my desire to teach!

"Doctor, can you check this lump that we found a short time ago. There's been no change in it at all recently." My first question is always, "Did she show it to you or did you find it?"

A lump that produces a limp or in some ways attracts the interest of the pet would be classified as an active one and should be operated on. The "found" lump should be closely monitored at home and only removed if:

1. A change, larger or firmer, occurs.
2. The pet becomes attracted to it.
3. A groomer irritates it during styling.
4. It is located on an eyelid margin and starts to irritate the cornea.
5. It's convenient, which means another procedure is needed that requires anesthesia.
6. "Aunt Ethel had a lump that was cancer and looked just like this."

Related to tumors, I actually coined a medical term which should (could maybe) make it into the next edition of *Stedman's Medical Dictionary*. And that term is "burywith." (It may be hyphenated if you like: "bury-with.")

A burywith refers to a growth that is nonclinical, having no justification whatsoever to be excised. The client is often overwhelmed when the term is used to describe a lump on her beloved pet. Any number of responses may be witnessed.

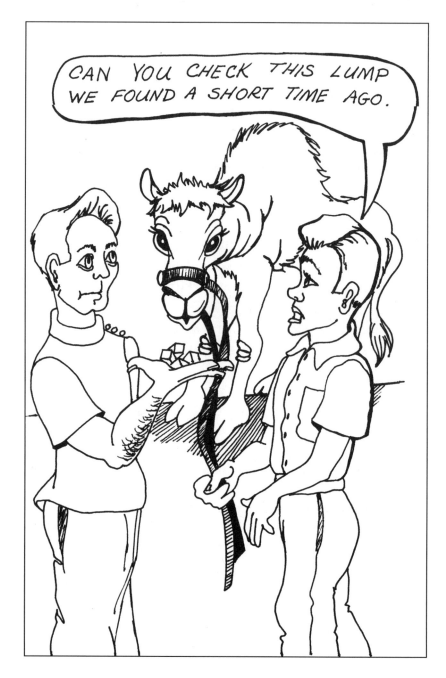

Disbelief, consternation, sadness, relief and then, "Just what is a burywith, Doctor?"

Joy overwhelms the room as I pronounce that a burywith is a growth that will accompany your pet to her last day on earth, and she'll be buried with it. No risk, no cost, whatta veterinarian!

A general surgeon at a local hospital now uses the term in his office, something his wife, also a client, relayed to me one day. I have a strong feeling he doesn't tell them the true origin of the word.

I learned — almost the hard way — that small dogs can be very protective even if their owner is a 250-pounder who doesn't need it. As I walked into the exam room, I recognized this ex-high school footballer standing at the table with "Peewee," his eleven-pound Pomeranian.

I tapped him on his upper arm so as to shake hands and, with that, Peewee took exception and attempted to put his teeth into my palm. He always was before and afterward an exemplary patient.

The act of touching means different things to different creatures. To people, namely Bobby and me, it was a sign of ongoing friendship. To Peewee it was an act of aggression towards one of his possessions.

In the mid-sixties a tiny, vibrant Boston terrier pup was presented for his initial visit. His joy was evidenced by his stubby, pig tail that wagged his body from the rib cage back. As most veterinary staffs love the breath of very young pups, I knew that these little ones liked our breath also.

I leaned closer to this fellow's face, and in one quick motion he turned his head and snagged the septum between my nostrils. It was indeed a misplaced lick delivered with needle-like fangs and not his tongue! Involuntary tears streamed down my face unbeknownst to the owner — not from pain but because of my sympathetic nervous system reaction.

As I raised my face to the client, my wet cheeks were obvious to her by now. I told her that I was just remembering "my happy days with Grammy who had a Boston terrier just like this one." My client bought my story hook, line, and sinker.

I literally could not touch the tip of my nose for two weeks.

A young lady came in with her two dogs for routine visits. Her thirty-pound chocolate poodle was delightful during all aspects of his physical exam, including the drawing of a blood sample from a front leg. He loved the touching and the attention. After he received his vaccines, I placed him on the floor. "Pierre" was the model patient.

But then there was dog #2! "Don't forget, Dr. W., that 'Brownie' doesn't like to be picked up. She'll struggle but won't bite." I successfully cradled Brownie in one arm and turned 180 degrees to weigh her, working the scale with my free hand. In those days we had no walk-on scales. Brownie acted annoyed and yipped a little.

Hearing Brownie's yip, the now "piranha" poodle leaped up and placed her fangs into my left buttock. I immediately

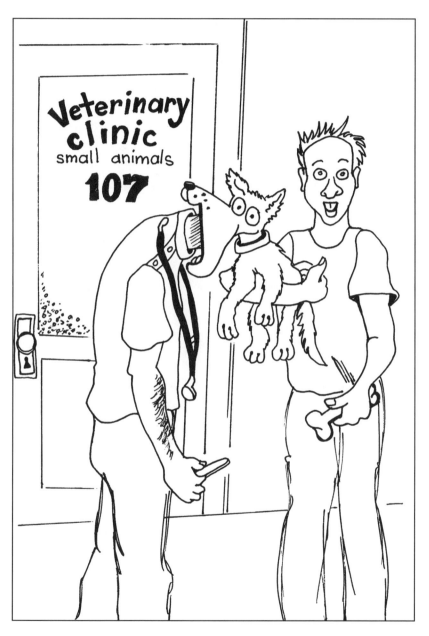

Most veterinary staffs love the breath of young pups.

became aware of a warm, wet feeling as I felt a tear in my trousers.

Since I was seeing this case at the satellite clinic on our home property, I excused myself and walked across the yard and into the house to change my slacks. With some difficulty I placed a Band-Aid on the inconveniently located punctures. Attired in new pants, wearing a smile on my face and enduring an uncomfortable bottom, I returned to finish Brownie's exam.

Whether it was because I was a too proud male, fearful of my registered-nurse wife waiting to explore the site, or just plain embarrassment, I chose *not* to discuss the incident that night after work. The next morning sitting down at the breakfast table was an impossibility. That night my wife inquired as to why I was taking a bath and not the customary shower. After my veiled explanation, I heard, "Okay, hold it. Let me examine your wound."

Now nurses have a reputation of being well-trained, very able, kind and considerate. This is not necessarily so with their husbands. The now exposed wound revealed that some skin had been forced into the underlying tissues and soaking would be beneficial — but not before the area had been thoroughly scrubbed and the inwardly deflected skin manually exteriorized to a more normal position. All this was accomplished by the aforementioned "gentle" nurse wife. Whatta a pain in the butt!

I was a young practitioner when an elderly beagler who, upon hearing my "don't-feed-your-dog-bones" lecture, said in rebuttal, "I've never had a problem in fifty-five years with my hounds." (He had that "you young whippersnapper" tone of voice.) I amazed myself when I replied, "Then you've been lucky for those fifty-five years."

If your dog dies from eating the bones found from a dead bird or opossum, that's bad. But it's not quite as bad as if you had fed him a pork chop bone yourself. Sure, you get the same result, but the psychological difference needs no explanation. I can recall doing a rectal exam once and seeing blood on the *inside* of my glove — *my* own blood! It was the bones in the dog's rectum that cut my finger. You can imagine the damage that could be inflicted on the dog's GI tract, and those of us who have had surgery "there" appreciate the potential for pain.

And speaking of surgeons, allow me to explain how I lost a client forever. A woman brought in a new beagle-mix puppy that was happily awaiting my entrance into the exam room. "Mrs. Surgeon" persisted in referring to her newly obtained pup in the masculine gender.

To save time during an exam room conversation, a veterinarian will often keep eye contact with the client, maintain conversation, and let his fingers do the walking. Killing two birds with one stone is a great time saver. I discovered with this pup, oops — no scrotum, no testicles, no prepuce.

I subtlely inquired if "Mrs. Surgeon's" previous pet had been a male. She said, "No," and inquired as to why I had asked. A lot of people do call small pups "she" and larger ones "he." For that matter, to some, all dogs are males and all cats are females.

In this case, "Pickles" was a female. A look of total disbelief engulfed her at the sound of, what she considered, my totally misguided statement.

"My husband is a surgeon on the staff of XYZ hospital, and he has examined Pickles," she exclaimed with a presumptive attitude of "that should speak for itself!"

It certainly doesn't take a rocket scientist to differentiate a female from a male. Clearly, she was one off!

My next move apparently caused her to leave my practice forever, never to be seen again. Cradling the pup in the crook of my arm, I drew onto her lower abdomen, with a soft tip marking pen, the necessary, albeit missing, male paraphernalia.

A veterinarian had better know his audience well when he teases a client by saying that "living in squalor allows wax to form in their pet's ears." Or to the chagrined owner of the stool-eating dog, when he says, "It is an excellent form of recycling and it *is* cheaper than dog food." Or, "When the door opens, disease walks in and veterinarians are there to fight it."

It takes three attributes to be a good veterinarian, and they are: good looks, intelligence, and personality. Isn't that obvious? You'd better know your audience very well when making these tongue-in-cheek statements. I've certainly had to relearn this lesson several times over the years.

"Bailey" is a golden retriever who, because of her youthful personality and extremely small size (only 55 pounds), would have made a young veterinarian assume she was only six months old until her owner said, "She's six." But I've known Peggy for thirty some years and Bailey for all six of hers. When

I say this dog has a youthful personality, I mean exuberant! She greets her veterinarian on only two legs, jumping forward with front paws extended waiting for the hug. . . and treats.

Since I have had both of my knees replaced, this form of greeting from one of my favorites puts me in a tenuous position. Though my incisions are long healed, I've become predictably overprotective of my scars. So when Bailey came for a recent visit, I walked into the exam room with my back turned to her and Peggy. Then I greeted them with my neck turned around about 90 degrees. In actuality, I was cautiously protecting not just my two knees but a third area of my body (too personal to mention), which had been at peril because of previous greetings by happy canines that day.

When you set serious goals, always make them attainable. Unrealistic ones lead only to frustration. Let me elaborate.

On the top of every patient file is a space reserved for important data. This would include medical information, such as dosage for long term therapy (epilepsy, cardiac, diabetes), drug reaction history, and persistent personality traits. The latter is a kind way of saying what size muzzle to use on a dog or if protective cowhide gloves are required for a specific feline.

Wonderful pets are so noted here also. And on extremely rare occasions not only does the patient receive the highest of accolades but the client also. "Wonderful dog. Great family." One in five hundred, maybe.

"Gypsy" is just such a yellow Labrador. And her owner, an E.R. nurse, warrants high marks also. Recently it came time for Gypsy to have a new playmate. So a rottweiler pup was pur-

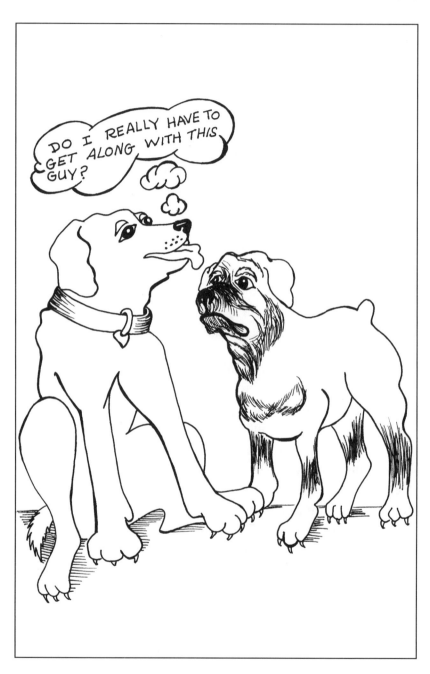

chased, introduced to her new household, and shortly thereafter presented for her first physical exam.

No Gypsy was he. Not even close! The shy head turn and the guttural sounds emitted during paw-touching told me to approach this pup with caution — not a good sign in a nine-week-old. The owner's immediate response was one of disappointment. Of course you could never compare this rookie to Gypsy. The contrast even made the rottie look worse since the aging retriever was a tough act to follow.

With a touch of embarrassment, Carol said, "Some day 'Morgan' will have the same remarks on his file also." That goal will be unattainable, I'm afraid. But he's off to a very good start.

This family has made great strides with Morgan to the point that he is easily managed in our office. And this is a compliment to our accurate description of "great family." But "wonderful dog?" Not quite yet, but getting close — very, very close.

"Mongo" was the first highly trained guard dog that I had ever met. As expected, he was a very large German shepherd — and what else would you expect with a name like Mongo.

Michael, whom I had met some dozen years prior as a blond, freckled-faced, ten-year-old lad, was now a uniformed member of a railway security team. "Doc, I don't want you to walk into the exam room while we're already in it. How about you wait in there for us to come in to you? This is precautionary; he's new to me also."

Over the ensuing years, the three of us grew closer and closer, even to the point of Mongo trusting me to cut his nails. I know he liked and trusted me as much as I did him. This is one of two M and M tales in this book. In this case, Mongo, Michael, and oh yes a third M, the muzzle.

Apomorphine is an extremely interesting pharmaceutical used only in dogs. Cats are very sensitive to morphine derivatives, and its use in felines can cause seizures. The drug is a highly effective emetic, that is, it produces vomition. Its use is specifically for that — to induce vomiting when indicated.

Years ago, veterinarians would inject a diluted amount of this pill after dissolving it. However, when vomiting was effectively produced, we couldn't suspend its activity, and sadly, retching would continue long after it was necessary.

Well, with all of today's research and technological advancements, we have an alternative approach, depicting just how far veterinary medicine has come. We now take a *chunk* (not a carefully weighed aliquot of drug, but a *chunk!*) of the same drug and place it on the surface of the dog's eye under its lower lid. When the desired effect is attained, the chunk is flushed out. (No, it cannot be used a second time. At least we haven't tried that yet!) This is a great improvement in a veterinarian's armamentarium.

A very recently engaged young woman was passing through our area and escorted her canine into our waiting room. "My dog just swallowed my ring and my fiancé is going to shoot me."

A quick x-ray confirmed her fears, the old ring-in-the-stomach trick. As a result, a "chunk" was plucked from a vial and placed under the eyelid, hopefully, to extricate the ring. Shortly thereafter, the aforementioned diamond, mingled with the delightful stomach contents, was on the floor.

One of our techs commented that it wasn't the size of the ring that counted but rather the love that allowed its purchase — one of the kindest remarks I ever heard her say.

People say interesting things about their pets!

"My dog doesn't need a leash; he's so well-trained." Yet, he would be the first one to jump onto someone walking by or lick another canine customer and provoke an altercation. And speaking of leashes, I'll never forget the client who hadn't realized her dachshund had walked out of its collar, leaving her to walk down the hall with a dogless leash. (That shows the value of a choke collar.)

"My dog would never bite." Everyone knows that if there are teeth in the mouth then the bite is available. However, I did lose a fingernail to a toothless terrier who "wouldn't bite." The gums were as firm as a tooth's enamel.

" 'Mikey's' panting so much, I'm sure he needs a bowl of water." Veterinarians are obligated to place the requested drink on the floor knowing full well that the drooling, panting bulldog is having an adrenaline rush and is just excited. One sniff is about all the water gets and deserves.

"My cat's heart is pounding extremely fast." The best answer after normal cardiac evaluation is that we get much more concerned if the heart stops. But we do ask the owner to check the resting rate at home and get back to us with that result.

Suffice it to say, a veterinarian's personality impacts a great deal on her "audience." With that in mind, it's my feeling that this trait is one of three that makes or breaks the client-doctor relationship.

First, if you are a personable doctor, people will want to return. Then if you solve their problems or do all within your means trying to do so, you will benefit. If it's obvious you love animals (and all people want you to love their animal family), this is the third piece of the puzzle.

Animal hospital employees who have all three are blessed, enjoy themselves and their jobs, and everyone around them benefits. Having any of the three attributes makes for success. But for contagious success, all three are necessary.

Shortly after the introduction of disposable needles and syringes, veterinary practices disposed of them as they saw fit. OSHA's appearance on the scene a decade later altered that to be sure. In order that "druggies" could not utilize this trashed equipment, we would snap off the hub of the syringe with the needle attached, return the needle to its plastic cover, and "hello" trash can.

One particular episode sticks with me on this topic. It involves an attractive client who came in without her husband. After administering the requisite vaccines for her West Highland white terrier, I smoothly and with a flair of coolness, snapped off the hub of the syringe while speaking of some important and current world situation.

Much to my chagrin the cool, one-handed snap allowed the twenty-two gauge needle to do a ninety-degree turn, penetrating the webbing between my thumb and index fingers.

I turned away saying that I hoped the shot didn't sting her Westie (anymore than me!). Deftly, I pulled out the impaling needle and set it on the sink counter.

To this day I don't know whether she thought I was kind and caring, incompetent, or oblivious to pain. The only hope was that she couldn't see what I could feel.

And speaking of accidental sticks, this story goes back to the pioneer days when veterinarians allowed owners to restrain their pets if they trusted them to do so effectively. "I can hold 'Barkley' for his rabies shot. I've done it before," declared Terry, a credible client and owner of this black cat.

The reaction was so quick on his part that Barkley's claw-filled left paw whipped back swiftly, surprising the "restraining" owner and whacking at my hand holding the three-cc syringe containing one cc of rabies vaccine. You just know what happened! The needle stuck my left index finger at the first joint. A droplet of the vaccine penetrated my skin.

I washed my hands, placed a Band-Aid on the site, and with technician assistance gave Barkley his slightly interrupted and momentarily delayed rabies shot.

About 3 AM that night, I was awakened by a throbbing of the "Barkley finger" where swelling had tightened the tape. The first thing I did in the morning was to call the pharmaceutical company that manufactured that particular vaccine. Because of a time zone difference, the extra hour only increased my concern. The anxiety was not for the inadvertent injection producing the disease itself but rather could anything else in it cause problems?

An hour later, I learned that St. Paul Ramsey Hospital in Minneapolis handled all accidental vaccine self-injections occurring in our nation. A knowledgeable, kindly registered nurse assured me that any worry would be related to the adjuvant or carrying agent which, in this case, was aluminum hydroxide.

None of the potential signs — swollen axillary lymph nodes or sloughing (dying skin) of my finger — ever occurred, but for two plus years the swelling remained, and my finger was sensitive to the slightest of touches.

Those touches always reminded me of that Monday evening way back when Barkley and I shared an injection. Barkley is no longer around, but the owner is as loyal as ever today. Maybe the several sleeves of golf balls I received over the years was a subtle apology to me. But their gift was never necessary as Barkley's family has always been and will continue to be one of our practice's favorites.

Certainly, most calls that a veterinarian receives during the wee hours are truly emergencies, and we have to bite the bullet when the phone rings. Long before an emergency center was opened locally, coverage was done on a practice-by-practice basis. That was difficult in itself, but especially so if several other practices decided not to respond to their own emergency calls, and as a result, their clients called me. It was not unusual to see fifteen to twenty of these cases on any given Sunday.

Our practice had always felt that if the client thought it was an emergency, then we assumed it truly was. And we trained our staff that way. So if the call concerned a cat that was seemingly screaming in pain, writhing on the floor seductively, you asked the obvious question, "Is your feline a young adult, unspayed female?"

If yes, we would merely tell the owner to call in the morning and make an appointment to have her spayed. Now if the pet had been a male feline, this meant the old "trousers over the pajamas, twenty-second teeth brushing dash" and a very rapid thirteen-mile trip to our hospital.

One of the very most common and serious emergency calls involves the urinary tract of the male cat. The same problem occurs in dogs. In the case of the dog, there is a more gradual onset and the call is usually made earlier by the owner. This emergency involves the pet that is unable to urinate because of a blockage created by an ongoing bladder infection.

People frequently witness their dogs urinating in the yard but rarely do they see their cats go to their litter boxes and perform. To many cats, it is a very private affair and I can relate to that.

Anytime an owner thinks his male cat is constipated, one must assume that the cat cannot urinate until proven otherwise. The inability to urinate is the most common killer of young male felines, more so than leukemia or road trauma.

Any animal that doesn't urinate for three days will die or "be at the door." Constipation is no emergency whatsoever. Some telltale questions that help differentiate the two would include: Is he making frequent, short trips to the litter box? Does he suddenly sit down to clean himself? Have you recently found urine in inappropriate sites?

Often cats with bladder infections (cystitis) will urinate in the sink or tub and blood is easily noted. Had he urinated in the litter box or on a rug it would not have been apparent.

The following cases are ones veterinarians agonize over but shouldn't have had to. The first was the client that assured me that his six-month-old setter mix could not get up and could I take a quick 2 AM look at him.

After my fifteen-minute drive, I was greeted by a family already in the parking lot. The young couple had a pajama clad youngster with them, and knowing that pediatrics was not my specialty, I asked the whereabouts of their close-to-death "other child." Just about then from the distant end of the parking lot appeared a happy-go-lucky tail-wagger.

"Doc, I guess she just wanted to get out into the fresh air. We don't owe you anything do we?"

"No, of course not." Some people!

The other emergency was the "no show" that I waited for nearly an hour. I called several times but to no avail. Finally I drove home and later learned that they had decided to call their neighbor whose veterinarian would be happy to see them at 3 AM and besides that she was closer. No call. No apology.

Fortunately, the opposite occurs on occasion. Here are two examples of overly kind, sympathetic caregivers whose sympathies were directed first toward their veterinarian instead of toward their pets.

It seems that the Willises had gone out for dinner and had left unattended the Halloween candy targeted for the next night's trick-or-treaters — close to three pounds of chocolates plus the usual other assortment. Unfortunately, "Toby," their coonhound, had helped himself to all of it. "We knew that chocolate was toxic but didn't want to disturb you after nine o'clock at night, Doctor," explained the Willises.

Biting my lip, I told them that veterinarians are on call to help their clients and be available to them and their pets. Of course, chocolate can be toxic but the situation could have been handled differently and quite possibly, Toby's death averted. Naturally, I said nothing about this in our conversation.

The second incident involved an elderly gentleman with his overweight chow. He arrived a half hour early for his late afternoon, mid-August appointment and told our front office staff that he'd wait in the car so as not to upset "Khan" or put pressure on our staff.

When his appointment time arrived, our receptionist went out to the vehicle where Mr. Handwerk was holding his hand to his dog's nonbreathing chest. "You know he'd been panting all day long and we hadn't gotten him shorn yet this summer. Heck, I even had to stop mowing this morning because of the humidity."

Heat stroke comes seasonally in our community and must be anticipated with certain breeds, especially when obesity is present. Shade, shade, shade. Water, water, water.

When the mowing became hazardous because of the heat, Khan should have been in the house with his master — for both their sakes. Again, the latter words were not uttered to this client who did not want to interfere with our schedule. Emergencies are our business — saving pet lives is what we strive to do every day.

While on the subject of emergencies, Bernice called early in the morning to announce that one of her schnauzers, "Adolf," was acutely ill with bloody mucous escaping rectally. A quick, presumptive 2 AM diagnosis of hemorrhagic gastroenteritis (HGE) was made. This syndrome, not uncommon in this breed, is fairly often brought in as a true emergency because of its signs and rapid onset. These canines are usually presented in shock-like states and must be treated both quickly and aggressively.

Blood samples were drawn for morning testing and, through the same intravenous catheter, steroids were introduced and fluids attached to run for the next few hours.

A possible etiology for HGE is thought to be an allergic phenomenon. This seemed quite plausible as all three had dined on veal earlier that evening, and I'm certain there were no leftovers in *that* house. This source of meat had rarely been included in their diet before, so the conclusion was logical. That being said, we were a bit more interested in Adolf's quick response to the intravenous steroids than playing Sherlock Holmes in the wee hours.

But something was amiss. Throughout that night's emergency visit, I kept hearing the off and on honking of a car's horn, but Bernice seemed oblivious to the sounds. My look of consternation evoked this response from my friend in her nasal voice, "Oh that's Nipchin, I left him in the car and he has no patience. He keeps beeping to get my attention."

Fortunately, like most veterinary hospitals, our practice was located in a nonresidential area. And I was hopeful that no security guard in this industrial neighborhood would be disturbed by the sound.

A young couple came in very distraught. They were sure their five-year-old spayed female Old English sheepdog had gone blind overnight.

I had to agree with their home diagnosis as I watched the gentle lamb-like pet wander into various items placed in the middle of the exam room. A cursory exam of the eyes revealed no abnormalities, and there was a positive reaction to a bright light. There was no obvious answer from me, so intravenous sedation and a more thorough ophthalmological exam was suggested that again yielded no helpful information.

The owners agreed to a referral to the University of Pennsylvania Veterinary School where one of my professors still taught and practiced. Early the next week a relieved couple related to me that "Princess Margaret" had been "cured and was back to normal."

It seems they had taken her to a new groomer the previous week, and instead of using a barrette to pull back her bangs, she combed them down over Maggie's forehead, unwittingly covering her eyes.

Later the referral letter from the University of Pennsylvania read in part, "Gene, you always gave the impression you had paid attention in class." After that, whenever I met my former professor, he would just shake his head before shaking my hand.

One does not place English bulldogs high up on the canine S.A.T. (intelligence) charts. However, it takes a modicum of intelligence to be vengeful.

When necessarily "inflicting" pain on a patient, a veterinarian might expect a reaction to the applied noxious stimulus, perhaps a turn or a vocalization: growl or hiss, a snap, a bite, some urine. These pets do not turn the other cheek.

Having completed the routine visit with the physical exam and the appropriate vaccines given, I walked past "Waldo," the bulldog, held on the table by his 275-pound owner. My graceful steps were just close enough for the semi-restrained dog to try to hurl himself off the table to attach himself to my arm. His forward progress was impeded, thankfully, by his master who was obviously used to his dog's tactics.

"Don't worry, I have him under control. That's just Waldo being Waldo." The client went on to relate that even at home he was a challenge to all except for very close family members. (Was the owner just trying to make me feel better?) When giving a party at their home and no matter the guest list, the owners put this muscular beast in their locked car parked in the locked garage. Let's hear it for safety!

At least the family knew their pet's personality. Vengeance is mine saith the bulldog.

The mother of one of our veterinary assistants brought her cat in for a routine visit. This well-tended Persian had as beautiful a personality as its coat, but it lacked something. She didn't smell like a cat but instead like heavy-duty smoke. If there is anything fortunate about a pet's shorter life expectancy, it's that they don't suffer the consequences of secondhand smoke so much in the news these past few years with humans.

With my nose in close proximity to "Toby's" long coat, I gently alluded to my olfactory sense findings. "That's it! Cheryl has been telling me about that for some time now. I'm quitting." And quit she did, at least till after she lost her Persian. I always wondered if she went for a coat-free pet next like the Chinese crested, Mexican hairless, or the sphinx cat — or did she remain really cigarette free?

A well-coifed toy poodle was being admitted for dental prophylaxis, and as Betty walked by with "Fifi" in her arms, she said, "Get a whiff of this one." Now Betty has been with my practice for over two decades and when she talks you pay attention.

Assuming she wanted me to identify the source of Fifi's odor to be Canine #5 or her mistress's Chanel, I came in direct contact with its hair with my ample-sized nose. As I hoped for Shalimar's or Jovan's musk oil scent, instead I was greeted with Marlboros or Kents — quite a let down.

Later that afternoon Betty discharged the stylish poodle postsurgically and received from the owner a smiling apology for her pet's nicotine odor.

"I guess you talked to the boss on the phone after her procedure this morning," Betty said.

"Oh yes, and I was so nervous I had a cigarette in the car on the way over. I'll never smoke again," the client answered.

Sure. At least she'll give it up once a year when Fifi comes in for her checkup. I have the strongest of feelings that her next two poodles smelled the same.

"Shamu" has been part of our practice for over nine years. He came along as excess baggage with one of our young veterinary associates. A client easily talked the recent graduate into finding a home for their nine-month-old, black and white, domestic shorthaired cat. This inexperienced, well-meaning veterinarian would find out soon enough in his career that pet doctors are frequently asked just that by clients — to place their beloved pet into a wonderful home. The owner often "forgets" to mention that the dog is a biter or the cat doesn't utilize his litter box. Neither of these criteria fits this yet-to-be-named feline, however.

It was a Monday morning when, much to my surprise, I met this skinny youngster for the first time. News of Shamu's arrival had not reached me, and as the owner of a thirty-member practice, I was quite disturbed not to have taken part in the decision-making process to keep him.

Before I had the opportunity to discuss his presence with anyone involved, my receptionist asked me to return the call of a client who had just hung up as I had arrived at the office. Although it was just shortly after 7:30 AM, I knew the client would be available.

"Hello, Mrs. Schmoyer, is 'Lilly's' back acting up again?" I started to ask. As I uttered those words, our newest "staff member," Shamu, in full purr, walked across the telephone keypad and disconnected us.

Love starts in many, many ways, and this was certainly one of those moments. I hugged this cat as I redialed to re-inquire about Lilly's back. Was it true love or just a subtle suggestion to start using a portable phone?

Clients have become accustomed to our ample-sized, grown cat and frequently ask for him. Regarding his weight, he is the classic example of "don't do as I do but do as I say."

Yes, Shamu bears that name in recognition of his body's conformation — svelte he is not. But lunching staffers rarely ignore his food seeking antics so dietary indiscretions are not uncommon.

Our clients often will say what a "big-boned" mascot you have, knowing the sensitivity our practice has for overweight pets. So Shamu continues to lie on our countertop on his short forays outside the staff lounge. And as far as I know, he never disconnected another call. He had accomplished what he desired with that initial *faux pas*, probably a well-thought-out plan.

A vocation that gives joy and excitement can create a positive force in life that is often contagious. That's what the exam room does for me.

Whether the situation is routine or dire, there are opportunities to create lasting bonds during a pet's visit to the animal hospital. This is a time to listen to people and their pets — a time to learn how to provide the type of atmosphere that minimizes stress and builds trust. Some days things seem to go as smooth as silk — but that's just some of the days!

CHAPTER IV

"Doctor, Is It Serious?"

"Maggie," my sixteen-year-old schnauzer friend, will die before you read this. She's the third schnauzer I've shared with this family. Stephanie was her current caregiver. She had lost her father four years ago and her mother two years later. I had known Stephanie since her teen years, and tears streaked her face as we reminisced about her parents and about Maggie's condition.

Recent setbacks had cost Maggie the good appetite she had maintained throughout her life. So I suggested that anything from the table would be in order. "Are you serious?" Steph retorted with good-humored sarcasm. "That's all our schnauzers have ever eaten all these years!"

No one in the family had ever admitted to me these ongoing dietary indiscretions on their pet's behalf. "Maggie loves fish and chicken but spaghetti is her favorite," Stephanie admitted. "Every time she eats marinara sauce, she has to rub her whiskers across the rug. Her least favorite food is chicken, but since we know it's healthier than beef, we 'force' her to have it on Mondays."

Later that week Steph called to let us know that Maggie's appetite was 80 percent back to normal. The 20 percent deficit was on Monday with the chicken entree that failed. "I broiled three pieces of chicken breast fillets but she rejected them," Steph reported. "I left them on a paper towel near her water bowl. I returned from work only to discover that she had deposited a B.M. on top of them."

I suggested she add marinara sauce next Monday.

Allow me to devise for you a pet first-aid kit for home use. It should include the following:

- rectal thermometer
- aspirin
- kaopectate, and
- a wrung-out washcloth kept in the freezer or a bag of frozen peas.

Frozen peas have been surprisingly effective for canine patients with bloody noses — an application much more acceptable to them than the time-honored ice pack — and for my own aching knees.

When we have allergies, the signs we manifest include: itchy, watery eyes, sneezing and a runny nose. Our allergy symptoms are associated with the respiratory tract; our pets, however, have dermatological signs evidenced by itching, licking, rubbing, biting, and scratching. The amount of histamine released is much greater in our pets than for us. This is the reason why antihistamines work wonders for us but just don't do it for our pets.

To give a pet allergy relief, a drug with potential side effects — prednisone — must be administered. Used judiciously, this steroid has tremendous anti-inflammatory capabilities and many, many valuable uses. The important word here is "judiciously."

As I explained previously, cystitis is a urinary tract infection evidenced in every animal species. It is also potentially the most common killer of young adult male cats. In felines, urinary bladder infections often lead to microscopic crystal-like formations in the urine which can precipitate together, form plugs, and prevent the passage of urine. Because of the anatomical difference between the sexes, urethral blockage occurs in the male cat but only rarely in the female. Understanding the behaviors and potential risks of this condition are terribly important, so I'll revisit the signs here.

It is difficult to discern whether a cat in its litter box position is urinating or defecating. So if a client calls and states that her cat is constipated, the veterinarian will ask two questions: "Do you have a male or a female? And are you seeing urine being passed?" Because the inability to urinate means life or death to the cat, it must be seen. And there is no choice in this matter if the call concerns a male. Constipation can become a complicated issue but not a particularly acute one.

Certainly, astute owners will take note of their pet's behavioral changes long before the late stage of straining to urinate occurs. These signs would include frequent trips to the litter box, sudden licking of the groin, and inappropriate urination.

What is inappropriate urination? It is small amounts of urine not within the confines of the litter box. And if these are tiny amounts, you wouldn't even be aware of them because of evaporation. The inability to detect the problem can be a serious situation. But by some quirk of their discomfort (possibly feline to man communication!), cat's frequently select the sink or bathtub instead of the litter box. On a porcelain or stainless-steel surface, blood in the urine is readily identified — a much easier (and preferred) detection spot than the oriental rug in the living room.

Most feral felines take a very long time even to become pettable. Sometimes it requires a *"cat*-astrophe." A family related such a tale in the office as they placed a cat, engulfed in a towel, on the exam table. They had been feeding this large fellow outside all summer, and he had still not overcome his extremely shy nature. Maybe, just maybe, it had something to do with their seven children and two dogs that made up this wonderful family.

Today's visit was prompted by a cat fight where, at the very best, he tied for last. Yes, he was pretty beat up! I don't know who adopted whom, but the adoption was complete as this new loyal feline is now overwhelmed with both human and canine love.

"Rosie" had a similar history with our own family. Rosie was a farm-born kitten who was "adopted" by us to provide rodent control for our farm — one whole acre including a house, barn, large chicken house/garage, and a two-seater outhouse (seldom used except for sudden emergencies — male only). So Rosie's domain was neither complicated nor far-reaching.

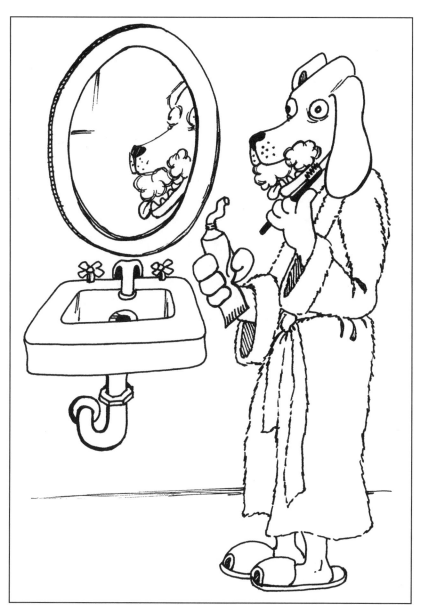

***Owners must
keep their dog's teeth clean.***

Of course, we expected to do nothing more than feed her and, in return, have mice delivered to us. Three weeks into Rosie's "probationary period," she was not to be found. Then one morning we heard a weak, baleful crying from underneath our barn overhang. Ironically, the exit door of our satellite clinic was located there. For the very first time in her life, Rosie accepted human hands. Extreme salivation and an asymmetrical face made it obvious that she had endured head trauma with a resultant fractured mandible (broken lower jaw). We supported her with fluid injections for several days and then softened food.

Shortly thereafter we introduced soaked kitten chow, and ultimately, dry food for the next fourteen years! She purred constantly (I could never adequately evaluate her heart over the purring) and she always responded, in kind, to our calls. Oftentimes I recall seeing Rosie lying on my wife's back while she was on all fours working in the flower beds. Rosie never grew to more than six and a half pounds, and I think most of it had to be heart.

With people, brushing our teeth is so important that this routine becomes quite automatic. After all, they're our teeth and we want to keep them. Veterinarians also advocate daily home dental care for pets. But periodically, when brushing my own at bedtime, I realize that I had forgotten "Sara's" and "Sophie's" teeth. "I'll do it tomorrow," I'd say and I would.

I keep their "doggie" toothbrush and toothpaste on the dish drying rack in our kitchen sink because I have nightly kitchen duty. Now don't think for a minute that the dog's don't enjoy this daily routine because they do. One famous bribe and reward method works beautifully for all breeds, but especially for our Labradors.

Give one-half dog biscuit before brushing, leaving the second half on the counter as an anticipated post-brushing reward. That's all that is required for this fifteen- to twenty-second procedure. In the end, people and canines are both satisfied.

So when a veterinarian proposes to clients that dental care begins at home early in life to control bad breath, don't expect dental prophylaxis under general anesthesia to resolve that problem except temporarily. I speak now only of your pet's bad breath.

Dentistries will specifically improve the oral health of the pet as well as its overall health in the long term. But brushing and more brushing will always maintain the results gained after you've invested in a veterinary dental procedure. Not uncommonly, an owner will call back two months after a dentistry to tell us that her fourteen-year-old cocker is acting like a new dog. Now that's a fringe benefit to help make a veterinarian's day.

July 4, 1963, sticks with me as a day of personal infamy. I was a virtual infant in practice — one month — when an eye-opening experience taught me much about love or lack of same.

The emergency call came from two elderly sisters who presented an equally geriatric Scottish terrier who had "developed bad breath only yesterday," they said.

A cursory exam revealed an oral cavity that overcame me. My first reaction was, "How do I not vomit?" Strands of mucus held a few premolars to the gums, and these were raw and oozing blood. I extracted all the remaining fifteen to twenty teeth this poor fellow had, some requiring my fingers only. More time was spent flushing the oral cavity than doing the extractions.

Seemingly, the wave of a syringe of sodium amytal (anesthesia) in front of the dog's face was enough to keep the dog comfortable during the short procedure. During this period in practice, this drug was the most commonly used for procedures of this length. I related this case because the two owners acted as "surgical assistants," and believe me, not of their own volition. They learned firsthand (hand's on!) what they had put their "beloved" pet through for months and months on end. Love is sometimes blind but should never be foolhardy.

Many people, of course, dislike it that general anesthesia must be utilized for dental prophylaxis and will, therefore, put it off as long as possible, and in many cases, too long. Inexperienced veterinarians, all too often, want to please an owner and sometimes agree to see "how things go" when it comes to dental care. It took me many years to realize clearly that what's best for the pet is best for the owner, despite their sensitivities. These pets were suffering as the result of the short-sightedness of their owners and their worry over anesthesia — rarely was it about the cost. Henceforth, I proposed mouth work in a more aggressive fashion rather than using the subtle approach of the "good old days."

What changed my attitude and my approach was twofold: an improved anesthesia protocol, namely isoflurane gas, and the one-month, post-prophylaxis telephone calls from clients telling me of the tremendous improvement in their pet's general demeanor. "I guess 'Julius's' mouth was worse than we thought." (Have you ever had a loose tooth? Been there — done that — over a one-year period with a failed root canal and six visits to an endodontist, which led to ultimate extraction and eventual resolution.) I could empathize.

Shelties and collies, more so than other breeds, not uncommonly develop a huge matting of hair behind and below the ears. These wads can actually twist down to the skin, and any indiscriminate use of scissors by a well-meaning owner could lead to veterinary surgical intervention — specifically, sutures to close an unfortunate laceration.

Careful use of an electric clipper is a safer way to go about removing matted hair. Once the areas are relieved of those wads, the following instructions are "my guarantee" to avoid recurrence: "Spend a total of ten seconds a day with a comb used at each shaved site. Starting today, you must do it daily for the next thirteen years. You'll never have another mat."

The reality is that the caregiver is likely to follow my instruction for only two to four weeks. The following year's visit generally proves my point; self-discipline is not easy. Maybe that's why we have Labrador retrievers and not collies!

When on call in the early days of my practice, we always spent social time with the closest of friends where we were within walking distance of the practice. This was long before the dawning of veterinary emergency centers. This particular Saturday evening was no different. As we shared an "apartment dinner" with friends who would eventually godparent our twins, Hal offered to accompany me to our office after the answering service advised me of someone with a cat in labor.

Hardly had I finished shaking hands with the client when the words, "It's not my cat," were uttered. The necessary ovariohysterectomy — rather than a Caesarian — was performed. Needless to say, that was one of my first experiences with the "never-to-be-paid" emergency visit so common in the veterinary profession. I was surprised that the "new owner" retrieved his "non-pet" that Sunday morning. But you never say "no" in such circumstances.

Pearl's sister-in-law had a rather large springer spaniel. We always treated and examined "Conrad" on the floor, not the exam table. He weighed ninety-four pounds! Since most veterinarians are kind folk, we often carry bags of pet food to someone's car, hold their babies, and the like while clients are finishing up at the desk. Today was no exception as I offered to walk Conrad out to his vehicle while his owner was paying her bill. "She belongs in the back seat," the elderly owner said after a sincere "thank you."

No sweat for me — six-foot-two, one-hundred-ninety-pound athlete that I was. But Conrad was difficult to boost up onto the backseat. His resentment was only expressed by a look of disapproval, but my brute strength was enough to overcome this weighty spaniel. He just did not want to get into the automobile.

I returned to the clinic, said my goodbyes, and started an office visit on a cat. The owner of the aforementioned pet returned to say that her Conrad could not to be found. "He must have escaped from my car." I quickly learned that the 1988 green Buick was not her blue 1980 Oldsmobile. I had put him in the wrong car — no wonder he seemed so obstinate when I lifted him into the back seat.

What would the scenario have been if someone had driven off without noticing him in the backseat or if he had paid me back by soiling the interior of that car? To this very day, as I continue in my gentlemanly ways, I have the owner give me their keys, an in-depth description of their vehicle, license plate and location. A gentleman surely. A dummy, unquestionably.

Feline owners without a cat carrier will often express concern about their trip to the veterinarian with a loose cat in the vehicle. We would often recommend a pillow case for the safety of all involved.

A client presented her pillow-case-confined cat to our practice, and of course, was asked if we had advised her of this method. "Yes, but I had some forebodings about its safety, so I walked around my apartment for an hour with a pillowcase secured over my head to convince myself."

Can you imagine the look on the face of the telephone repair person stopping in to check the apartment's phone service.

"My veterinarian told me. . . ."

"Yeah, sure lady, whatever you say."

New to practice and wanting to be all things to all people, I offered to return a schnauzer pup postsurgically to the owner who would otherwise have picked it up the following day. At the time I was driving a five-speed VW Beetle that obviously necessitated use of the clutch. This situation required a pet carrier but there was none readily available for this pup.

Allowing my heart to rule my head, I transported this free-roamer in my tiny car. Never again. One arm reaching across the passenger seat to contain the little guy worked fine until shifting gears was required. Hum, no third hand was available. Within seconds, the "wiggly-one" was exploring his new world of pedals. Driving on a busy interstate is bad enough, but with this distraction it was nearly impossible and certainly unsafe.

Life's lessons are often learned the hard way. Fortunately, nothing traumatic happened to either pet, driver, or vehicle. Suffice it to say, it was a very nerve-wracking and extremely slow twelve mile drive.

During the 1960s a family brought in their two pointers and a basset hound. All three were shy and distrusting pets. The family was seemingly very normal with the husband a corporate vice president and his wife a counselor. Or was it? Are three maladjusted dogs from the same family simply a coincidence?

During the reign of the third dog, I learned one of their cats had had a litter and kittens were available. Coincidentally, our management consultant and good friend, Dawn, was seeking a new feline companion. The veterinarian go-between strikes again!

I drove to and visited with the litter owners. It didn't take very long to understand the reason why the three canines had the personalities they had exhibited over the past decade.

It started with the slammed front door and continued with the constant attention seeking by three young children, ending with a loud and shrill, "WILL YOU PLEASE BE QUIET!" from their mother

I left their home with a changed attitude. Obviously, the environment here contributed greatly to the makeup of their canine charges. I crossed my fingers hoping that the kitten's "rescue" came before too much "emotional" damage had been done.

A veterinarian should never spay a stray female until it's proven she hasn't already been done. If you know she's a stray, has been a "rescue" for six months, and hasn't gone into heat, then you know *not* to do an exploratory. Usually you are able to discover a scar with shaving and alcohol application to the mid-abdomen. But not always!

Now if you don't know that the female is a stray, the picture changes. This question should be posed to the new owner prior to surgery. The ultimate responsibility certainly belongs to the surgeon. But if the system fails, it does so because of a string of failures from the front office, to the veterinary tech, and ultimately to the doctor.

One morning in my operating room, a forty-five minute "spay" revealed no reproductive organs available for removal — they were long gone. A "during-the-procedure" phone call gave us the requisite answer — a stray! "Oh, Doc, we forgot to tell you she was a stray." No, *we* forgot to ascertain this fact.

In our lifetime we will likely outlive five of our beloved cats or dogs. And we would agree that to have one of our children predecease us is life's worst nightmare. None of us ever wants to experience this, and our hearts go out to all our friends who have been through it.

This certainly is not meant to belittle the importance of our pets, especially to families who have not had the experience of parenthood. Too often we hear about the horrors to which pets are exposed. Unfortunately, people treat other people in like fashion, as our media informs us daily.

When love and caring are missing in a pet's life, as in a person's, that in itself is unacceptable. But worse than that is the abuse that can and does take place. Pet abuse needs to be understood to be stopped. The dog tied outside, fed once daily, and never routinely given a tender pat of kindness experiences a form of abuse. We rarely hear about this common situation because the headline-grabber is usually the pet maliciously shot or beaten.

We know that people often hurt pets because it hurts those who love them. So someone will kick the dog to "punish" a child. It's been demonstrated that abused pets live in homes where child or spouse abuse is likely to occur also.

The Pennsylvania State Veterinary Board no longer recommends the reporting of probable animal abuse cases to local authorities. It now *demands* it. Now it is not only morally and ethically a veterinarian's responsibility, but it is also a legal one.

We have a wonderful laminated pet "eye chart" that most clients understand is meant to be tongue-in-cheek. That is *most* people anyway. As I've said before you must know your audience.

The two-part chart depicts five levels of objects decreasing in size and increasing in numbers. The feline side starts with one large fish skeleton and ends with seven mice. The canine side

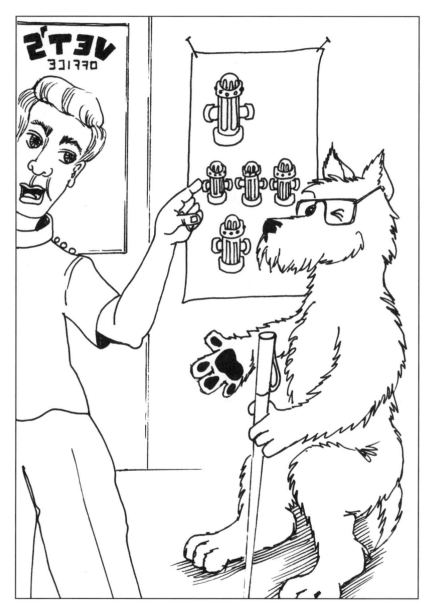

Even with only one eye,
Twinkle could still ace the eye chart.

starts with one large fire hydrant and ends with eight doggy treats.

When the client has a vacant stare as you hold up the chart for their pet, you know full well that you selected your audience poorly. That client's first question is: "How can you tell?" and then trails off as you quickly don your stethoscope and place the chart on the counter behind you.

Years ago, and to a lesser degree today, pet stores would have toy breeds flown in from around the U.S. for sale. Most of these dogs are bred in large puppy mills in the Midwest. Many of these pups are eight- to ten-week-old toy poodles, Yorkies, Maltese, and the like that weigh less than two pounds.

Chiefly because of size, age, and travel-related stress, these puppies would be carried into the office looking close to death, and certainly some were. They had infantile puppy shipping fever — IPSF (my coined name for an old disease).

This situation calls for immediate response. Shaving the neck and applying alcohol to find the jugular vein precedes the introduction of a tiny needle to administer the needed drug — 50 percent glucose (thick sugar water). These pups, more often than not, literally wanted to leap off the table as you carefully apply firm thumb pressure on the plunger of the syringe to have the thick syrupy fluid flow through the tiny needle's diameter. In these situations, veterinarians are heroes to the pet shop owners, and the veterinary staff is as proud as peacocks for this timely, lifesaving opportunity.

Another opportunity for instant heroism would involve the female whose recently whelped pups had rapidly depleted the "milk-shed" and now the "ole gal" lies on her side seizuring. (This condition would be the equivalent of milk fever seen by large animal practitioners.)

Again the use of an intravenous drug produces Herculean effects as the grand mal seizuring lessens. The patient goes gradually from stiffness to relaxation, makes a conscious effort to right herself, staggers for several moments, shakes herself awkwardly with wagging tail, and says, "Bring on the kids!"

This powerful drug is calcium, a mineral that has been stripped from the dam through the milk taken from her to nourish those newborns. How mothers sacrifice for their children! As opposed to the glucose treatment mentioned earlier, calcium must be injected slowly while monitoring the heart rate. Its rapid infusion will cause bradycardia (decreased heart rate) creating the potential for an orphaned litter. The veterinarian again becomes the momentary champion to all present — owner and staff.

Judy and Fritz came in with an adorable three-pound dachshund who was as cuddly as any of her predecessors in this household. A distinctive feature characterized her as very special. "Heidi" had a right-angled tip to her tail. The last inch-and-a-half formed a perfect L. We all agreed that both for health and aesthetic reasons, the last two inches of her tail should be amputated at the time of ovariohysterectomy.

Later that day, our close friendship necessitated my personal involvement with Heidi's discharge. The tip of her tail hung over my shirt pocket as Julie handed them their pet. Their thankfulness for the success of the surgery was brightened more as laughter followed. They did not want the souvenir to take home. Definitely another case of know your audience.

A common complaint of pet owners is this: the toe nails are too long. Certainly long nails will have a greater tendency to break or snag on things. Only occasionally will the dewclaw (thumb) actually become ingrown.

Any incident involving toenails can be painful and may require sedation to be remedied. Having had an ingrown nail in the distant past, I can relate well to the sensitivity of this portion of our anatomy.

Getting a new pup accustomed to paw playing is beneficial in future years because they will accept nail trimming more readily. In senior dogs, altered gait is often blamed by the client on overly long nails. Not so. Arthritic joints lead to a breakdown of these joints, and the dog is no longer able to walk "proud" but rather down on their pads, often referred to as flat-footed. This will allow the nails to become excessively long and not wear down. Some will actually become entwined with the adjacent nail. Thus the overgrowth is the *result* of joint breakdown rather than the opposite.

Another common complaint is self-interest in the dog's own hindquarters, be it actual rear end dragging or licking itself near the tail base. This is usually the result of impacted anal glands and not worms as often thought by owners. A distant second cause would be fleabite allergy.

Anal glands are analogous to the scent glands of skunks whose use for protection is familiar to all of us. The odor of the expressed substance is musk or fish-like and it "stays with you."

When a veterinarian cleans the anal glands, the exhaust fan is put on high, and the owner given the opportunity to exit.

When teaching owners who want to try to resolve this at home, remember two things — do so outdoors and no peeking.

And here's why. Years ago, an attractive client's Great Dane was exhibiting the usual signs of rear-end dragging, spontaneous licking under the tail, and the characteristic odor of "Mr. Yuck." I wisely went outside with both of them to empty the culprits with glove in hand. Fortunately, it was a gorgeous day at the satellite clinic adjacent to our house. Coincidentally, my wife was walking out to pick up the mail. Timing is everything. She gave me one of those "what's-he-up-to-now" looks. Joan had obviously not seen my glove, only an unescorted lady and the Dane who outweighed her by more than twenty pounds.

When I did the rectal on this gentle Dane, I wisely stood off to the side, not directly in line with his tail. I proceeded to apply increasing gentle pressure to the left gland and "milked" out its contents into the appropriately placed wad of cotton. The right side was a different story. The ghastly material exploded just over my shoulder, hitting our pioneer fence some twelve feet to the rear. Always stay out of the line of fire!

Later that day my wife told me that she only believed my tale of the tail after she had checked the fence.

Another source of odors would be the pet who rolls on carrion — the remains of another animal. They also gain pleasure by turning onto their side, rubbing shoulder first into excrement. Mother Nature has provided the canine with the ability to disguise its own scent to discourage predators. But that Good Mother doesn't have to live in the same house with said beast to share its potent "eau natural" cologne.

These distinctive odors can best be neutralized with a combination of one quart hydrogen peroxide, 1/4 cup baking soda, and 1 teaspoon of Dove dish soap. This recipe also serves well the ubiquitous skunked-dog syndrome. One hour after applying the mixture to all affected areas, the preparation should be rinsed away. I pass this knowledge on as a personal success story.

My wife was in the backyard one summer night with our black Labs when she noticed "Sara" paying more attention than usual to our barbecue grill. It didn't take long before a one-pound, "baby" skunk crept out from underneath the grill stand and did his or her "thing" into the face of our very surprised Lab. Without delay, I mixed the ingredients of my "famous" scent-removing concoction and sponged the patient thoroughly with it. Owing to the lateness of the hour, I deferred rinsing off my "magic potion" until the morning.

Well, the next day, Sara was relatively odor-free to our delight — but she had also partially taken on the appearance of a Chesapeake Bay retriever since her "peroxided" head bore striking brown highlights, a symbol of her skunk experience that lasted for nearly four months. She'd become a marked canine in more ways than one!

I very often tell people whose pets experience excessive itchiness that it's like you or me with poison ivy. When we have it, the more we scratch it, the better it feels, the worse it gets, and if left alone, it will start to remedy itself.

Because we cannot give twenty-four hour supervision to our pets, specific oral medications are prescribed. Why do these pets seemingly scratch more at night? That's easily answered. During the day there are many distractions — children, TV, radio, phone calls, mail delivery, traffic, and daylight. The itchiness is as profound but interest is easily redirected.

People will call up to complain that they were told by one of our staff that their cat did not have fleas. What she should have heard was that no fleas were found. If you see a flea, then you have fleas. If you don't, then it means you *probably* don't have fleas.

Why do fleas hang out on our cats and dogs, ignoring us? Body temperature. Because we register on average 98.6 degrees normally and our pets are about three degrees warmer, our friendly insects choose Florida's beaches over Alaska's mountains.

You've heard the saying "like rats leaving a sinking ship." When veterinarians administer anesthesia, the pet's metabolism slows thus decreasing body temperature. And if the sleeping furred friend has fleas, well, they're like the rats. They scurry for the warmer environs of the sleeping subject, like under the tail or scruff of the neck. And we'll have the opportunity to witness this not uncommon migratory pattern.

Flea eggs remain dormant over the winter while cold temperatures kill off the other stages of their life cycle. Interestingly, we've seen wildlife roadkill brought in for disposal that are carrying live fleas. So if your pet is out there with recently dead animals in the middle of winter, don't be surprised if you find one or two fleas. Even after a killing frost, we'll see flea outbreaks one to two weeks after a period of so-called Indian summer.

While on the subject, there are two ways to determine if you have those "dreaded" fleas in your home. Let's assume that you're going away for an overnight with your pets and your house is totally animal free (except for the fish in the aquarium) for that period. Upon your return, leave all pets in your car and then enter wearing shorts and be barefoot.

Fleas will be seeking a food source — your blood — and since you're available, even your "lukewarm" body, to them, is better than no meal at all. Additionally, if your spouse hangs out in the backyard while you bring in all the luggage, well, maybe he or she is smarter than you think.

The second method for flea discovery applies when there are no travel plans in the near future. Take a gooseneck desk lamp and bend it down as close as possible to a saucer with dish detergent in water. Place this scientific piece of lab equipment in the most likely flea area, for example your pet's bedding. Then leave it turned on overnight.

If present, the critters will do a cannonball into the concoction and drown. You not only identify a curable/controllable situation but also have established a nonpesticidal method of control. It could be termed flea suicide.

An elderly disadvantaged woman placed her toy poodle from her lap up onto the exam table and asked forthrightly, "Do you remember me?" The assertive attitude was followed by equally aggressive placement of a puppy booklet next to her pet. It was a brochure that we had utilized before 1970 and, therefore, had not been seen for thirty-some years.

"You haven't changed much young man except for the gray hair. You wrote some notes in here more than two decades ago, and I want to tell you a few things about yourself." This peaked not only my interest but that of three staff members who overheard her loud observations.

"I'm a handwriting expert frequently called upon by government agencies to evaluate personality via the written word. If

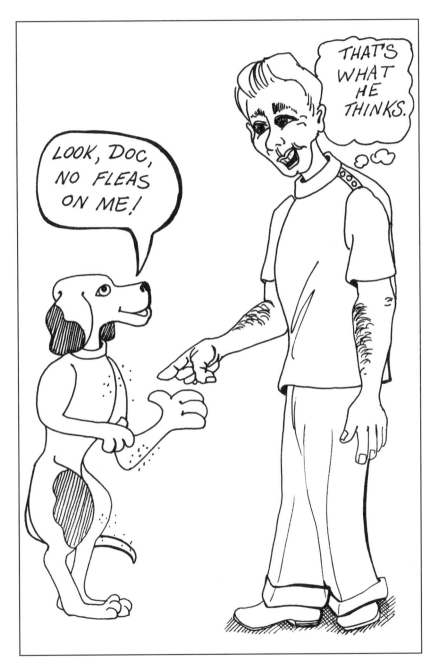

you're ever in need of an after-dinner speaker, just call me and I'll guarantee you good entertainment with my unbelievable accuracy."

She blew me away when she opened the puppy pamphlet and I recognized my cursive writing way back when. "You are capable of being interrupted in mid-sentence, excuse yourself and then return minutes later to finish that sentence. You can also count pills and write on a record while holding an intelligent conversation on the phone."

To my amazement she was very accurate, and my three nosy veterinary assistants cracked up in delight over her comments. Maybe all veterinarians have this ability, because one tries to be all things to all people at all times.

Because of the high esteem the medical profession deservedly receives, I always felt it to be a wonderful compliment when a pet owner would say, "We wish you were our family's doctor." We all agree that bedside manner, or in this case, cageside manner, is so very important. I've wondered at times if the true family doctor is ever told the reverse, "We wish you could be our veterinarian."

CHAPTER V

Children and Their Pets

Kittens, puppies, infants and toddlers. What do they all have in common? For starters, they are young and extremely dependent on their parents. Our four-legged youngsters are used to *maternal* leadership and very little, if any, nurturing from the male side of their heritage.

To a veterinarian, those young felines and canines are the future of the practice. But vastly more important are those children who truly hold the future of our profession in their tiny palms. They are the generation that will provide a loving home for their family pets today and will bring us their own pets tomorrow. That said, it never hurts to start developing new relationships at an early age! So I say to the young mother, "May I hold your baby while you take off your coat?" Or to the cute toddler, "Give me your hand and I'll show you some other puppies."

I never miss an opportunity to apply a tongue depressor splint to a teddy bear or a bandage to Raggedy Ann's injured elbow. But each child must grant me permission to do that — and they often won't! After all, it's *their* baby and they are very protective. So those moments are between the child and doctor. The parents simply look on!

Art Linkletter, a pioneer TV host and author, wrote a book called *Kids Say the Darndest Things*. As you may know, his TV show had the same title. In the veterinary office the opportunity for a child with a pet to say something "memorable" reinforces Art Linkletter's theory. What those kids say may be *very* personal. Take Timmy, for instance.

Timmy was sitting on our scale when I asked this two-year-old how he was feeling today. A few seconds passed, then he looked at his mom and said, "I just farted." Lucinda and I will never forget those words, and, I'm sure, for years Tim won't be allowed to forget them either.

"What's your pet's name?"
"Where do you go to school?"
" How old are you?"
These questions to a youngster are a quick way to get to know a family in the exam room. When children are present,

they get my attention first — the parents just need to wait a bit. And they never seem to mind. A big handshake for the young caregiver and a big "thank you" to them for bringing both their pet and their parents for an office visit will generally evoke a memorable smile.

Addressing remarks on feeding and training to the suitably aged child will underline the importance of pet-care responsibility and teamwork at home. Many times children are the ones expected to shoulder these requirements, so why shouldn't they be the ones who get the veterinarian's attention?

Another way to get children interested in their pet's health care is to get them involved during the visit. I often have them help me determine their pup's weight. Obviously, the child's age and ability are also considered before we start.

First, I write out the following equation:

Dr. + Pup = 206 pounds
Dr. = 196 pounds
Pup = ? pounds

After we calculate the weight together, I give the paper to the child to take home. It could end up on the refrigerator!

Whenever I've spoken to scout groups or at an elementary school, I have left knowing that these future pet owners have learned five important points.

1. Never handle a wild animal.
2. Never feed a bone to a dog.
3. All pets must be spayed or neutered.
4. Never allow your pet to get fat.
5. The most important part of your pet is its leash.

I usually ask the leader/teacher to ask their children to submit a question in writing ahead of time. That's my way of trying to include all the youngsters and to "honor" even the shyest of the shy. By explaining these five points during the presentation and allowing all the children to become involved, I am always touched by the proudly raised hands at the end of the "lecture."

As payment for my efforts with these young animal advocates, each is asked to send me a note explaining what they learned. The innovativeness of these notes is extraordinary, and these moments are another one of the fringe benefits of my profession.

An analogous situation to Darwin's theory of survival of the fittest is the creation of what is known in nature as the "pecking order." In graphic terms this means, "Down on the farm, let's see who gets to eat first in the chicken coop." What many parents and children don't realize is that there are pecking order issues when a new puppy comes into the household.

When a new pup is introduced into a family setting, he tests everyone around him, not only to establish his identity but also to seek his place in line — his "pecking order" position. He will challenge Father whose stern, deep voice he quickly respects; mother's role is also valued as a higher authority; a teenage caregiver will likely reinforce the rules, but the four-year-old toddler, last in line, is an easy mark for puppy pushiness.

The pup will play with the toddler and dominate him as his newly discovered "littermate." This is noteworthy because of the love they'll come to share and just how much each of them lets the other get away with. Most significantly, theirs will likely become a "win-win" relationship.

Teaching children not to feed table foods to their dogs takes some doing (although it is often less difficult than teaching some adults the same thing). One set of parents told me that their dog had developed diarrhea attributable to a hand-feeding child. The child was then taught that it was his responsibility to clean up after his dog, inside or out. These were caring parents who took the time to teach their youngsters this valuable lesson which will be a lifetime benefit.

Jenna was a lovely youngster who wore her emotions on her coat sleeve. "I love you, Dr. Witiak." Those words, impeccably pronounced by this three-year-old, were as honest as they were sensitive. The openness and candor of children makes everything more meaningful and important.

Besides being adorable and well-mannered, she brought a freshness to our office and had me looking forward to their visits. We see even more of their family now as they are keenly involved with the Siberian husky rescue group.

Every visit required me to pick Jenna up and carry her around our hospital to visit other pets and people. Whenever a day is going poorly, I recall those moments when I transported that sweet young lady in my arms with her head pressed against my chest and her arms lovingly around my neck. That memory always brings a smile. I'm sure I will be retired from practice when she's a knock-out college cheerleader — but you never know!

Some children, however, are brought along to the veterinary office when a suddenly sick pet requires an unplanned trip. Because of the unavailability of a baby sitter, two youngsters trudged in with their mother, adding pressure to all involved. Their boredom became obvious shortly after entering the exam room.

The four-year-old walked behind me as I started to examine "Tigger." Her brother stood on the chair behind his mother. A loud sound caused me to turn my head to see the daughter opening and slamming shut the cabinet door beneath the sink. After several moments of silence from the parent and growls from the feline, I suggested she might correct her daughter.

"Oh, this is your house and you should administer the discipline."

By this time I had walked behind the seemingly oblivious mother — not to give *her* the deserved correction — but to rescue her son, "Tarzan," from his precarious chair-top perch. It was a test of patience all around.

From the mouths of (older) babes came the following:

"My dad lost his two favorite girls within the same year — our dog died and I got married."

"When I graduated from college, my father gave me luggage."

"My kitten is sick and won't eat. Well, ever since we shared a tuna salad sandwich last Wednesday she won't touch her kitty chow. And she keeps following me around."

"We always thought 'Thelma' would be a great name for a kitten. It didn't matter he was a male."

I met fourteen-year-old Tyrone for the first time when he came in with his uncle who was also his guardian. Tyrone was large for his age but in a healthy way. In his arms was the most loved toy poodle pup you ever saw.

Uncle Steve explained to me that Tyrone had been in a snowmobiling accident the previous year. His lengthy hospital stay was due to a head injury that left him in a coma.

He abruptly "woke" and shortly thereafter began rehab. I was fortunate to meet him during the time that both his physical and psychological traumas were healing.

Tyrone had been "kissed by an angel" — that sweet toy poodle that Steve acquired from a friend. Little was known about this curly licker who brightened the eyes of this nonsmiling young teenager. There seemed to have been many burdens on Tyrone during his youthful years.

It just so happened that the "selected" date of this toy pup's birth was the same day that Tyrone woke from his coma and became aware of his surroundings. That birth date discussion also brought a look (though barely perceptible) of joy to Tyrone's face. I'll never forget that visit.

M&Ms have always been a favorite around our practice, especially during the Easter season. When a young lad accompanied by his mother entered the exam room eating a packet of those chocolate delicacies, I, of course, commented, "I see your mom made you a well-balanced lunch today" — tongue-in-cheek, of course. I mentioned that I too loved those delectable, colorful treats.

"I even eat them in my mashed potatoes, and my mother puts them in my scrambled eggs," I jokingly told them. This brought forth much laughter but more importantly for the next five years or so, they gave me a bag of M&Ms each visit — for my scrambled eggs and mashed potatoes, of course! Actually, I prefer them straight out of the bag.

Weekly, one of our veterinary assistants brought her three-year-old daughter to our satellite clinic in the morning where her mother-in-law could pick her up for the day. On that day, Grammy was delayed about an hour because of a grocery store detour.

A normal three-year-old's attention span can be expanded only for a short time. One new puppy wellness exam followed by two feline castrations was not enough to keep her interested. So a tired boredom began to put pressure on the entire staff, including her mom, as the toddler sought her own avenues of interest.

My suggestion — intended to be both fatherly and kindly — was to have our largest stainless steel cage well-blanketed and then to place the tiring beauty in for a nap. Then when Grammy arrived, we escorted her to the dog ward to retrieve her precious one! "I wish I had my camera," she quipped.

Now I'll jettison back thirty years to recall our own family in a similar situation. Picture our twin daughters of infant-seat age called out with their parents to perform an emergency Caesarian section. I had been a solo practitioner for three years and not infrequently needed family assistance for night calls. More than a few clients who came in contact with the entire entourage still comment on it years later.

On one of those occasions we decided to bring along a camera. Well now, the photo of our daughters sleeping in infant seats in a thirty-six inch cage with the door closed did not sit well with their grandmother to be sure.

Our daughters were five years old when the "Ernie" story happened. He was one of three barn cats we had that helped control the mouse population on our property. That particular night I had left to pick up the babysitter. In the few minutes it took to deliver the sitter to our home and pick up Joan, Ernie had been hit and killed by a car at the end of our driveway. It was obvious by his appearance that he had suffered little.

Knowing our children would want a burial, we planned one for the following morning. I placed his body in a pillowcase prior to the graveside ceremony. Fighting back tears, we bravely broke the news to our twins.

"Can we see him please?"

"Yeah, yeah," was the supporting sister's response.

A quick look into the pillowcase revealed Ernie's face and neck, about the only parts that appeared normal. The glance satisfied their interest. Tears misted over the parent's eyes as the four of us pitched some of God's good earth onto the pillowcase carefully laid in the freshly dug grave. Parents just *know* when they are needed for hugs and understanding for their saddened children in precious moments like this, or so we thought.

We waited for grieving and crying, prepared to mix our tears with theirs, and the usual "he's with God now in the great SPCA in the sky." As we watched closely, our older twin elbowed her sister saying, "Well, that takes care of Ernie. Let's go get our bikes."

Just whose shoulder was for whom?

Children and their pets have a special relationship — one that we as adults may never fully understand. They may be drawn to each other because of their innocence and curiosity or by their desire to need and be needed. Whatever the reason, each pet will have an effect on the child's life, and most likely, their relationship will also be a family affair.

CHAPTER VI

If It's Not One Thing, It's Another!

A number of years ago, an elderly couple, loyal to our practice, would bring me their two Scottish terriers for their care.

On this particular visit, their older Scottie was the subject of attention. These conscientious owners wanted me to remove several innocuous skin growths, moles in actuality, that either bothered "Mollie" or were irritated during grooming and would start to ooze.

"Fine," I said, "and while she's under anesthesia, we can do some dental prophylaxis to improve her oral hygiene."

I suggested that, while pre-op testing was being finalized overnight, the owners map out on four 3 x 5 cards the location of each mole. Each of the cards would cover a major specific body surface. The reasons for requesting this activity were twofold:

1. Help reinforce the sites I had previously recorded.
2. Give them something to do to "help out" — to be involved.

The day of surgery arrived and we were presented with one Scottie dog and four beautiful renditions of left side, right side, top and bottom. But instead of showing the six growths we had discussed, they had identified *twenty-two* for excision.

Following the induction of anesthesia, the surgical sites needed to be shaved and vacuumed prior to moving Mollie to the operating room. One veterinary technician started the shaving process and soon a second clipper joined in. As carefully as possible they buzzed away. Each growth required a minimal amount of hairless skin for surgical prep.

The problems arose immediately when the shaving revealed many early stage moles that were inadvertently nicked, were also in the surgical fields, and oozed. What was intended to be about forty-five minutes of anesthesia turned into almost two hours. Needless to say, Mollie's breath problem was not remedied as we postponed her dental care until a later date.

A total of eight sites actually needed excision with sutures; the other sixty-eight required electrocauterization — a total of *seventy-six growths* were removed!

This experience taught me to beware the elderly couple with little to do but present drawings in minute detail of their beloved pet companion prior to surgery. Now when they come in annually for routine care, they start by saying, "Do you remember Mollie and. . . ."

Our now infamous black cat named "Jasper" was the reason I married my wife (more on that in Chapter 10). The three of us met in 1960 when he was converted to a gentleman from a prospective streetwise gigolo.

Several years later Jasper developed a rodent ulcer, which is an area of ulceration on the lips. Back then, this syndrome was thought to be related to excessive licking and treatment was extremely variable, meaning a permanent solution often was not attained. Whenever this was found, rest assured that no practitioner knew the true etiology. Today, we understand it to be an immune-related disease.

I had put Jasper under anesthesia five times for various procedures intended to resolve the problem, including both electrical and chemical cauterization, excision, and suturing. But these efforts were to no avail. All the responses had been short term; recurrence always followed.

One day a human dermatologist came in with his German shepherd and our conversation, for whatever reason, turned to Jasper's problem. He told me that radiation might be an excellent approach since everything else we had tried had failed. He offered his assistance and the capabilities of his medical office.

In those days our only means of lengthy (longer than a half-hour) anesthesia was intravenous sodium pentobarbital. Since I had to arrive at this doctor's office with a suitably sleeping feline, I administered the IV in our veterinary office, wrapped our "child" in a baby blanket, and hustled off to his nearby dermatology office.

Sitting in his waiting room, I sensed several patients staring at me and my bundle. As my name was called I stood up and realized why the people had been so attentive to my blanketed possession. Jasper's tail had been hanging out of his covering. As I recall their questioning looks, I imagined them thinking, "I wonder what his wife looks like?"

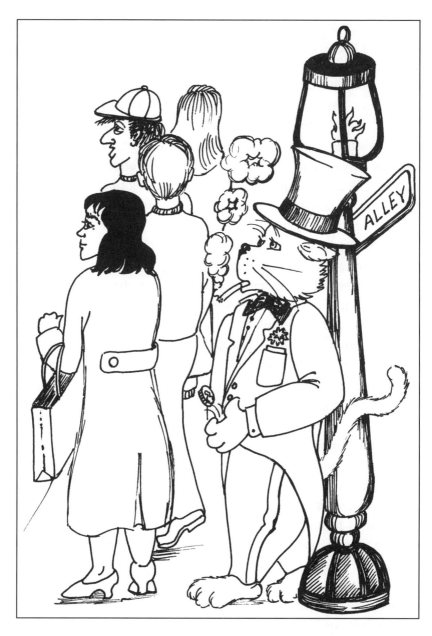

We saved Jasper from becoming a streetwise gigolo.

As it turns out this caper was worth the effort. The radiation treatment was a success, making Jasper a very happy cat.

I had just completed a cystotomy and a permanent perineal urethostomy on a five-year-old male English setter. Allow me to clarify. The dog in question developed urinary bladder stones of varying sizes, and in trying to urinate, several of these small calculi lodged in his urethra. Although the dog kept producing urine, he was unable to void because of the dam-like situation in his penis. And if one cannot urinate, one dies.

Today, veterinarians can remove the offending culprits from both the bladder and penile urethra, introduce a specific dietary regimen for the remainder of his life, and in most cases, prevent recurrent stone formation. Back in the "old days" these postoperative diets were only in the discussion phase.

Before the bladder stones were removed (the cystotomy), an incision was made through the skin covering the penis in front of the scrotum, exposing the stones in the urethra. This tiny tube, about the diameter of a Q-tip, was opened about three-quarters of an inch by cutting this "hose" not across but lengthwise.

Because the stones could recur, the incision into the "hose" was sutured to the skin on both sides along its full three-quarter inch length, thus forming an opening perhaps six to eight times larger that the normal opening at the tip. Thus a permanent aperture was made three inches from the normal site. This created a safer avenue of exit for the urine and any potentially formed calculi.

For several reasons, I personally discharged this dog two days postoperatively. This gave me the opportunity to promote the capabilities of my practice and also veterinary medicine in general.

Giving this owner a clear picture of all that happened afforded her the opportunity to ask questions. This was all done after the veterinary technician explained the preceding day's activities.

Now, there is a potential downside to this surgical procedure. The dog's new stream of urine can be slightly misguided because it has a new point of exit. So, as I stood on the porch of our hospital holding the dog's leash and discussing all the above, the owner interrupted me to point out that her recovering dog was marking a porch pillar, but its stream was running down the leg of my trousers. She said how embarrassed *she* was. How do you think I felt?

Twenty or so years ago, an oral antibiotic designed for the bovine species was introduced in liquid form. For years prior we used it in small animal practice for selective situations. Its use was not frequent because of the expense and because it was a capsule that many owners found difficult to administer.

The pharmaceutical representative called on us one day to recommend a new use for this now liquid antibiotic made for cows, even though our practice only takes care of small animals. (I'm at the point in my career when I have to ask if cows are the ones wearing the saddle or the ones bearing the large breasts!)

Because we liked this pharmaceutical "rep," we gave him his moment in the sun to tell us his recommendations for the use of this antibiotic. We all knew that dogs with a bandaged or splinted extremity would have a great tendency to try to remove it — lick, bite, chew.

"Doc, this drug tastes so bad that a dog'll never chew at it," he declared. Well, words are okay but I needed proof.

"Try it," he said, as I wafted it towards my nose. I stuck my pinky finger into the liquid and touched it to my tongue.

No amount of cold water rinsing followed by a mouthful of hot coffee afforded relief from the most bitter, horrible taste known to veterinary kind. The residual taste lasted well over half an hour. But knowing full well what animals eat or roll in for that matter, they'd probably enjoy this ill-flavored substance all the more. Our enthusiastic drug rep made no sale that particular day.

Owners are often concerned about the serious nature of anesthesia. And rightly so. But the stories they've heard should never prevent doing a necessary procedure that is in their pet's best interest.

Occasionally, I am asked, "Do animals experience cumulative damage from repeated periods of anesthesia?"

Because of the tremendous advancements in injectable sedation and oral narcotics we now enjoy in practice, the negative impacts of anesthesia are rare. Twenty-five years ago our only short acting intravenous drug was sodium amytal, a barbiturate. There are now better alternatives. In those years we had to do what we had to do.

A nine-month old German shepherd was accompanying its owner on a 150-mile trip from a central Pennsylvania town to upstate New York. For whatever reason he was tied to the bed of a pickup truck. This owner claimed to love to travel with his dog, his close companion! Really now! The blaring of horns drew his attention to the fact that "Prince" had fallen or leaped to the roadway and was dragged a short distance at 55 to 60 miles per hour. (Do you remember the movie *Vacation* and Aunt Edna's dog?)

Fortunately, he stopped quickly before a horrible death ensued. The dog's four paws were damaged; the injured front two paws, which were "skinned" down to exposed tendons and bone, were the result of the poor creature's efforts to stop the forward motion of the pickup.

For seven consecutive days, we anesthetized that dog for about fifteen minutes and three of us soaked, debrided, cleansed and wrapped all four of his feet. By the end of the week the two less damaged paws were doing quite well and would not require surgery. The front paws were certainly going to need it from someone more experienced than a general practitioner like me.

Our intention was to keep the shepherd stable and have the feet in a healing mode. When the owner made his reappearance to pick up his dog, he had his friend's station wagon for his return trip. I'd love to complete this story with a happy ending but there was no closure. No phone calls. No nothing, including the remaining 50 percent of his bill.

A moist eczema is an area on a pet's body that he self-mutilates by biting or scratching to the point that a raw, oozing "hot spot" is produced. No one knows what the causative agent is, but because most "hot spots" are seen in the hot, damp months of July and August, humidity is a probable factor. There is a breed predilection for this phenomenon — namely, the golden retriever in first place and the Saint Bernard a distant second.

If the site of annoyance is reachable by the mouth, then the tongue and teeth do the damage. But if not orally accessible, then the toenails produce the trauma. It's another one of those situations similar to you or me having poison ivy — the more we scratch it, the better it feels, and the worse it gets. If we would leave it alone, it would go away.

So a veterinarian will institute both topical and systemic medication to bring about relief. Sometimes it's even necessary to put the dog in an Elizabethan (no scratch) collar when you're not at home to supervise and distract your dog from obsessing about this annoying condition. An Elizabethan collar is a large circular plastic piece placed around a pet's neck and attached to its collar. It prevents the animal's mouth from reaching an incision or bandage.

Now, here's my worst "hot spot" case. Perma, an elderly woman who was our original hospital cleaning lady, brought in her Eskimo spitz because he was chewing at his tail. She warned me that her dog was extremely nervous and would bite.

Even before we attempted to place him on the exam table, he squatted, urinated, and in an act of frenzy, bit off three inches of his tail. As he screamed in agony, I saw the severed tail lying on the floor. (I never forgot that moment!) That afternoon I amputated his tail to about a two-inch length, and he never had a "hot spot" again. But he did remain a very irritable patient through his last years. His mistress kept us up-to-date about this rascal while she faithfully kept our hospital spotlessly clean.

Postsurgically, we often see our pets act out in one of several ways. The most common is, of course, "Hey I'm home from the hospital. Where are my toys and the food bowl." (In the case of the Labrador, reverse that order!) A pet doesn't become involved with its incisions as we do with ours. Now I must admit that pets will occasionally become spiteful after being taken to the boarding kennel or animal hospital, or they will seek sympathy for all the aggravation you caused them. In this way they certainly act more as we do under the same circumstances.

Experience tells us that an injured dog should be handled cautiously because even the kindest pet will bite if not carefully managed while in pain. Then there's the nasty dog that presents his aggressive disposition up front. Owners of the latter either are capable of assisting without putting anyone at risk, even to the point of bringing in their own muzzle, or cannot handle them at all, and we know where we stand with these dogs. (If our capable veterinary technicians are at risk, then drugs must be utilized.)

In general, people with big dogs usually manage them well. Conversely, in many cases, those four-legged friends that weigh less than twenty pounds, have lived a life on someone's lap, have self-determined their diet, and made their own rules at home, will get quite upset on the exam table when they are no longer in control. The owners of the latter either say, " I don't need help" or "He won't bite," which is not always the case since their dentition is still available.

You have to be able to differentiate between the credible client and the one who is embarrassed to admit that upon occasion his dog will show aggressive behavior.

Advanced age brings with it issues for both humans and pets. An example of "senior citizen syndrome" (SCS-human) is becoming more and more common around my house where I often find myself saying, "Why did I come into this room, anyway?" A client recently talked about her own "moments of anxiety" (MOA) and further related a similar situation of "senior canine syndrome" (SCS-dog).

Her aging companion had access to a flapped doggie doorway that gave him freedom to come and go into a protected backyard. In his very late years, he would go part way out of the doggie door, and for whatever reason — the weather or a siren — would stop in his tracks and have a bowel movement *inside* the house with his forequarters *outside* the house. ("Now, where did I leave my keys?")

People picture large breed dogs as being our main challenge. And believe me when I say that the large, truly aggressive canines are the most difficult. But when checking the temperature of a rottweiler or a chow, you're several feet from the teeth. They at least give you some reaction time. Not so with a toy breed.

The dogs that are most apt to harm someone are the ones with the Dr. Jekyll and Mr. Hyde personality. They lull you into a false sense of security, making you over-confident. Having confidence in your ability in any situation presents an illusion that you are in control, and this, in most instances, affects the client and the patient positively. However, over-confidence can lead the veterinarian into thinking that he can conquer all. And don't think for a moment that the dog doesn't see through this facade! The conqueror can quickly become the conquered.

One of our nicest pet owners had a ninety-five pound malamute. She always came in equipped with her dog's muzzle, and because of this, participated in office visits. This particular day, we all agreed that "Sheba" was in a submissive mood and didn't need to be muzzled. She rolled onto her back as I gently examined the minimal rash on her inner thighs. So far, everything was going along smooth as silk. She sat on her haunches as I started to place my stethoscope on her chest. Some inner voice told me to bow my head as I knelt next to her on the floor. With snake-like quickness, she snapped at what would have been my nose but instead removed a thin layer of skin from my then bloodied scalp.

Sheba had lulled me into that position of over-confidence. It was a setup. Who said dogs aren't intelligent? Guess who's always muzzled now?

Anytime you see a dog's tail pointing in the same direction as its nose, beware; you have a frightened canine that might not be trusted.

My first job as a veterinary associate was in a very busy small animal practice that also included boarding space for over one hundred pets. A very close friend of the owner would occasionally board her young unneutered male boxer there.

On one of their vacations he stayed with us for a week. During this period in the kennel he ate every morsel offered him yet lost close to fifteen pounds. Upon their return to retrieve "Ruggles," they could not understand how their beloved canine had been so neglected. They were quite angry with the practice owner in spite of their many years of friendship.

What they had not known — until they were so informed — was that poor Ruggles was mentally and hormonally involved with an in-heat boarding female, and it was difficult for him to sleep while panting with an increased heart rate and blood pressure. His testosterone level was also up — if you know what I mean!

Owners, like parents, are proud of their beloved pets and like to have them exhibit their abilities (and rightfully so). Rarely does a dog perform as well in our office as he does at home. So when I walked in to meet this springer spaniel for his annual visit, I was very impressed with the dog's response to its owner's commands of "sit" and "stay." And I expressed those sentiments exactly. The dog maintained his position but just couldn't wait to greet me.

After several seconds, his master "released" him from his sit-stay and he graciously approached while wagging his entire rear half. "Do you want to see one better, "I was asked.

"Of course," was my answer.

The owner told me to watch closely as he reached his hand into a pants pocket. His hand reappeared with his fingers formed like a pistol, and his voice made the sound of a shot. With that, the pet literally fell to the floor, rolled onto his back, and extended all four legs.

I immediately called Terry and Sherry to come in and witness this actor. They were veterinary assistants within earshot. The owner, with great deliberation and a very willing spaniel, repeated the performance for us all. I'm sure they remember that day very well even today.

A few years later, I related this story to a client who turned out to be a neighbor of this well-trained spaniel. Here I was talking like a very proud grandparent and it wasn't even *my* dog!

One of the most interesting learned activities performed by a dog at home intrigued me greatly, probably because it was a Labrador — an intelligent Lab at that. (Yes, that's an oxymoron.) The owner explained to me that before he left for work in the morning, he would put three treats on the hearth of his fireplace. They were spaced about three feet apart.

Apparently the dog would eat them separately, allowing a couple of hours digestion time between each. He had trained her on weekends and could therefore sneak a peak through a window to prove that she was being obedient. We never thought to attempt this one with any of our Labradors. We knew we would be doomed to failure.

Another client related a story about his two very intelligent Irish setters. Only one of them fit comfortably on their favorite sleeping site — the living room sofa. When someone rang the doorbell, they would good-naturedly run to the door, barking to announce that a guest had arrived.

Knowing the circumstances full well, the smarter (less dumb?) of the pair would bark and run to the front door while the other was, of course, enjoying the solace of the couch in pleasant slumber. The barking would wake the sleeping dog and cause it to leap from the comfort of the sofa in full bark and run toward the door.

But to his chagrin, not only was no guest present but now his warmed bed was occupied by his "partner." The instigator must have been a female who easily outsmarted her male companion. So what's so new about that?

Housebreaking is, of course, one of the most time-consuming, important aspects of a new pup's initial training. Like all veterinarians I stress that if a pup is unable to be supervised and must be left alone, then it cannot be allowed out of its "bed." This is best accomplished by "crating" which has become a popular and successful training aid for the past twenty or so years. Prior to its popularity, people believed incorrectly that this was a form of punishment. And in the very early days of practice, my thoughts were not much different. It didn't take much for me to become a convert. The crate's value takes on added significance when chewing things like furniture becomes a problem when many pups are between six and nine months of age.

If you don't have room for a crate or find them too costly, you can limit the pup to his bed in any of a number of ways. Try a cat carrier for a smaller breed pup or a piece of plywood triangulating a corner in the kitchen; some people will "short leash" their dogs to a radiator. The theory, of course, is that pups do not want to soil their bedding.

If the pup has the run of the kitchen and wakes up at 4 AM with "some needs," he walks as far from his bed as possible "to do it," and then returns to his sleep. If he awakes in the limited space of only his "bed" (the crate), then he'll turn over and go back to sleep and dream of puppy treats, postponing his potty needs.

If a young dog is purchased from a pet store, the situation is complicated since the purchased one has not been given any opportunity for early training. He has already been messing his bed (cage) which was not his fault, and your patience must be extended until he figures out what you expect. Success will follow from your praise and hugs. The good news is that this process gets easier with each succeeding pup.

Frequently a young pup doesn't know what the outside is for. New owners will walk the pup for an hour, play with her for a long period, tie her while leaves are raked, and the list goes on. If you want your pup housebroken, you must only take her out for two minutes, and if "nothing happens," back in you both go. Repeat this every fifteen minutes. On one of these trips she will defecate and/or urinate and your praises should flow. Give her the treat you always have with you — it's called your warmest hug — as well as the oft-carried food treat. *Then* return to the house.

The formula for housebreaking is a simple equation:

Understanding of Outside + Supervision Inside + Patience = Success.

Most clients express surprise when the newly acquired pup treats the crate as if it were a place of security when it ambles into it to take a nap. This doesn't happen overnight but patience always pays off. So have patience with the patient. It truly becomes the dog den or lair, a place to escape *us*.

We often hear owners say, "Oh doctor, she's only eight weeks old and we don't want her to get a chill by making her go outside."

In 1977 we had to house-train our eight-week-old, West Highland white terrier pup. She weighed in at a light three pounds. The lawn was covered by about an inch of snow that was capped by a thin crust that crunched under foot. The wind was howling at a severe 20 to 25 miles per hour.

I had on heavy boots and a hooded winter coat over my flannel pajamas as I carried this delicate, fragile pup outside. As I set "Twinkle" on the whitened grass, a wind gust blew her across our side yard on the thin veil of ice and onto my neighbor's property. That was a distance of about seventy-five feet. Twinkle still got the job done!

So saying "it's too cold outside" is not a valid reason to skip outside "potty time."

Let's for a moment discuss aesthetics and the veterinary practice. Specifically this subject will cover three topics: pills, stethoscopes, and ties.

Certain antibiotics come in beautiful, Crayola-like colors. Some examples would be hot pink erythromycin, the bright blue 100mg amoxicillin, its sister 200mg cranberry amoxicillin, and the senior size 400mg amoxicillin that is a fine green. I'll often tell the client that the medication may not work but at least they're pretty. One must be very selective about clients chosen to discuss pill efficacy versus their inherent beauty.

Stethoscopes also come in varying colors. You're probably more than familiar with the time-honored black models. Diversification has not only produced more aurally sensitive instruments but also ones less scary than those black ones: shades of grays, burgundy, teal and even a lime-colored version are available.

Frequently I'll enter the exam room wearing three or four stethoscopes and ask the client which goes best with my shirt and tie. They never pick the lime.

Speaking of ties, my daughters started buying me Snoopy ties for work since they are extremely colorful, in vogue for veterinarians, and have cool titles on the back. The tie depicting a canine Michael Jordan and all sorts of athletic equipment says, "I don't want to be an all-star, just a credit to my breed."

But my favorites are the Save the Children ties, which are a fundraiser for the foundation of the same name. These are neckties designed by children between the ages of five and fourteen, and are as diverse and imaginative as you would expect from kids in that age group.

Their uniqueness is exemplified by the fact that they most often depict varying professions that children love and respect, and in some cases want to pursue themselves. And what child doesn't love animals. So "our" ties — those veterinary ties — far outnumber any others.

Some excellent examples would be "Man's Best Friend," "Animals Love Ties," "Long Little Doggie" to name a few. And when I flip one over to share it with a client, especially children, you see the title and its "designer's" name. All eyes light up.

These ties are conversation pieces and are extremely colorful, so much so that upon occasion I have difficulty coordinating the proper tie with the proper stethoscope. Luckily, there's always that dust-collecting, black one lying around somewhere, and black goes with everything.

I've often said, "If the pets could come in by themselves — perhaps with a note tied to their collar — then everyone would want to become a veterinarian."

I've also said jokingly over the years that three attributes make a successful veterinarian and that would be good looks, intelligence, and personality. Truly, these *are* three qualities that separate the good from the best.

If a veterinarian is an efficient problem solver and a good surgeon, that's important. If he or she is able to exhibit a true love for each patient, that's special. Add to this an engaging personality and an ability to interact with the entire family, and that's the entire package.

If your veterinarian has any of these talents he or she is successful. A combination of all three will lead to years of pleasurable practice for both doctor and family. If you go to a veterinarian who doesn't see every possible upside to your beloved friend, maybe its time for a switch. A great partnership is a wonderful thing, and when it exists to serve the trusting creatures that serve us, the connection is more about love than science.

CHAPTER VII

Swallowed Objects

Any book on veterinary practice would be incomplete without reflections on "foreign bodies." When children are between two and half and four years of age, they will frequently pick something up and, if the size is right, put it in their nose or ear. (Their mouth is usually a distant third choice.)

My mother used to remind me that at the age of four, she took me to the hospital because I pushed a button up my nostril. Most foreign objects entering the body through the nose are, fortunately, passed in a bowel movement.

Why this tangential information? Well, a dog's fingers are its teeth. So when a dog gets its teeth latched onto selected man-made objects, not to mention some of Mother Nature's finest products, down the chute they go.

Twice I have seen a foreign object in a dog's oral cavity that looked like wound-up black thread attached to the roof of the animal's mouth or its tongue. In both cases, young dogs were presented with facial pawing, which was perceived as pain by the owner, or at the least, an acute annoyance. Both times the diagnosis was a well-attached carpenter ant that did not enjoy my attempts at its removal. The patient didn't like it either. Both retrievers required intravenous sedation to dislodge these critters. So beware the hidden dangers to dogs gnawing on old, damp wood — a favorite vacation spot for carpenter ants!

String or any thin linear material over two feet long is always a serious foreign body risk. If your pet is lucky, the swallowed yarn, string, leader line, or the like will pass straight through the GI tract relatively easily and end up on your grass. However, if that line becomes lodged underneath the base of the tongue and swallowed, it can cause serious problems.

Here's what can happen. While the animal is licking the stringy "object," it becomes wound around the underportion of the tongue and becomes balled up there. The animal's normal swallowing routine will then dislodge the string enough for the two ends to move into the stomach and then pass into the intestines.

Because of the string's entanglement at the tongue's frenulum (base), the two ends can travel no further.

Now the constant propulsive motion of the intestines — termed peristalsis — allows the string to take on a saw-like action against the inner wall of the bowel. This leads ultimately to penetration and then leakage of the bowel, causing peritonitis. Without an early diagnosis and rapid surgery, a grave prognosis will result in death.

Unfortunately, radiographs (x-rays) are of no value in the diagnostic process unless the swallowed line has a needle attached. This is the only time you would consider yourself lucky to have your pet swallow that metallic object, readily seen by the x-ray.

However, if the swallowed object is a large wadded up ball of linear material in the stomach, the results are only slightly different. A good example of this would be the cording used to wrap a roast or a ball of yarn. Because of its size, this mass may not be able to pass through the stomach, except for any loose ends that may be several feet in length.

The results are the same because the lower intestines again succumb to a sawing action of the immovable material. In addition, the peristalsis could cause an accordion or pleating-like effect on the bowel and ultimately lead to death. That's why these conditions warrant aggressive, surgical intervention.

In these situations, a skilled (and often lucky) veterinarian will smell a foul odor from the pet's mouth and may discover the string under its tongue. And if really skilled (*extremely* lucky), he or she will palpate the foreign body — the "accordion" — in the pet's abdomen. To any veterinarian, it's always better to have a negative exploratory operation than a positive necropsy (animal autopsy). In other words, finding nothing in a live animal is a whole lot better than discovering what the problem is in a dead one. So if your vet suspects this is what's going on with your pet, trust him or her to intervene with an aggressive move to surgery.

Other popular items that do not show up on x-rays but may be palpated would be plastic, corncobs, carrots, socks, and so on. It's swallowable if it fits in your pet's mouth. So if the clinical signs imply a foreign body, and an object not belonging there is felt, trust your veterinarian. Remember: a positive x-ray proves something is there, but a negative one does not prove nothing is there!

Foreign bodies that can be identified on a radiograph are termed radiopaque. These would include metal, bone, and solid rubber. These are no-brainers diagnostically and therefore will be operated on with more confidence since you pretty much know what to expect.

In our office we use a process that is often successful in resolving a situation where a pet has swallowed a needle or pins that are identified on an x-ray.

We take eight to ten cotton balls soaked in mineral or baby oil and push them down the pet's mouth, forcing them to be swallowed. When the cotton balls are passed in the next bowel movement, we check them for these pointy seamstress culprits. It works famously — again, if you're lucky!

Yes, if it fits in the pet's mouth, it can end up in the stomach. Case in point: In 1994 a four-year-old golden retriever was presented with a history of periodic vomiting over the prior six to eight weeks. An x-ray later that day revealed an interesting finding, which led to a phone call to the owner.

"Do you or your husband play racquet ball?" the veterinarian asked.

"Yes. Why? Did he chew one up?" the woman replied.

"No, ma'am," our young associate veterinarian answered. "He swallowed eleven of the balls whole and requires surgery to remove them."

Now these pieces of athletic equipment are made of solid rubber and make for a truly interesting x-ray picture. I never could understand how that many balls could be missing without anyone in that household questioning the situation. I guess it's just "easy come, easy go" for racquet balls among aficionados. It sure wasn't an easy go for their dog.

The same year, and only coincidentally, it was also a young adult golden retriever that came in with persistent vomiting. This situation had prevailed for six weeks and had gradually turned into constant overnight retching. This retriever needed two surgeries to remove some unique offenders it had swallowed. The first procedure removed 185 — by accurate count — one-and-a-half-inch long nails from the stomach. Three days later the thirteen nails that had been lodged in the esophagus (causing the overnight retching) passed into the stomach and were also removed.

Two separate surgeries were performed to avoid opening up his chest to access the esophagus. Chest and esophageal procedures are much more difficult to perform and the potential for complications much greater.

The source of the total of 198 nails, which weighed nearly two pounds, was the owner's basement workshop. Attempted canine suicide? Not so. Remember, this was a retriever. My suspicion is that while laying out some home improvement project, the owner stopped to enjoy a hoagie loaded with olive oil that may have dripped into the nail box. Overwhelmed by the draw

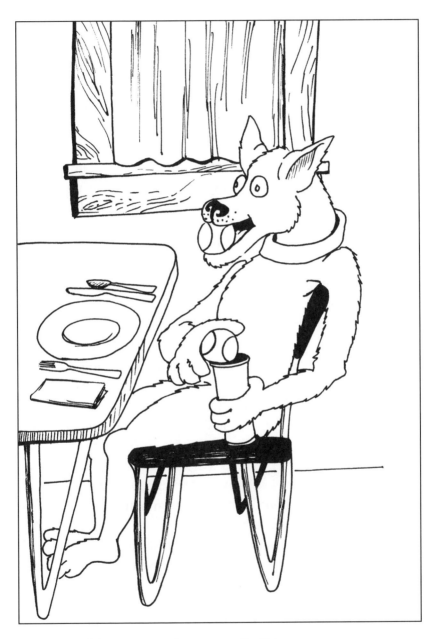

Next year at the racquetball tourney . . . .

of the "nail" salad dressing, this retriever felt compelled to eat what his master had eaten. I'm certain — positively — that this dog didn't chew each mouthful for the recommended twelve times before swallowing as we humans are encouraged to do. This dog gave a whole new meaning to the expression "sucking up lunch!"

I knew that fishhooks could be ingested, but fortunately, I'd never seen one go beyond the mouth. This one was impossible to forget. My fish story involves a lure called a plug, which is used to simulate live bait. At either end of the plug is a treble (three barb) hook.

A four-month-old mixed breed pup picked up one of these plugs in its mouth and hooked its lip on one barbed end. That was bad enough. The situation suddenly worsened when he reflexively tried to dislodge it with a front paw. Sure enough, the paw snagged onto the lure's other end.

The pup was now impaled and the harder he pulled his paw, the more his lip hurt and the more his lip hurt, the more he pulled his paw. I was thrilled to help this little fellow by administering an intravenous sedative when he first came in as an emergency. In a few short moments the situation was resolved. I was certainly not envious of the owner who had to drive to our practice with his pup crying the whole way. The sorrow felt both for the victim and the owner fairly quickly turned to joy and a sense of accomplishment.

A peach is a wondrous gift of nature only slightly improved by the hand of man and his ability to hybridize this fruit. But a peach pit in the stomach of a four-pound Yorkshire terrier is not a good thing.

In November 1983, Bill, who owned a moving company, called to say that "Misty," their one-year-old spayed female Yorkie had swallowed a peach pit. Now mind you, his was a *small* Yorkie. As difficult as this was to fathom, we still had to take the word of this insistent elderly man and his wife. To disprove this "impossibility," we examined their dog and took two x-rays, which revealed nothing which is what we expected.

Fifty-seven months later (just three months shy of five years), the same Yorkshire terrier came in as an emergency with very acute abdominal pain (a severe tummy ache). The blood tests did nothing to determine the cause of this extreme pain. Exploratory surgery was done immediately which revealed — you guessed it — that very same peach pit!

That not so tender morsel had lain dormant in the Yorkie's stomach for all those years. During that time the enzymatic activity in the stomach and constant mixing of its contents caused the pit to become both slightly smaller and very slippery. As a result, it was propulsed through the pylorus, exiting the stomach, to lodge in the small intestine. It got stuck there because its diameter was larger than the dog's bowel at that site.

The surgery was both gratifying and quick as this "freak of nature" was easily plucked from a half-inch incision into the duodenum. Fortunately, this fruit eater's demise was averted and she lived fourteen more years, proving once again that eating fruit promotes a long and healthy life!

I'll never forget October 10, 1972 at 8:30 PM. It would be the only time in forty years in practice that I would make it to the local emergency room for personal reasons. Sutures at the base of my thumb were courtesy of Mr. K's seven-year-old Saint Bernard whose name escapes me. It was the old "he doesn't like his feet touched but I can handle him while you trim his nails" trick. Veterinarians were more adventurous back in the "pioneer days" of practice — long before our litigious society pronounced veterinarians totally responsible for all persons participating in the management of their pet during office visits. This was both a hand- and eye-opening experience.

Bite wounds are at best an inconvenience, but because I was alone in practice at the time, I had to finish up about another hour and a half of appointments before my quick visit to the hospital. Another reason I can easily recall with great ease this client's name is because this very same "man-eating" Saint, when a ninety-five-pound six-month-old, swallowed a most interesting foreign object.

I was in a four-veterinarian practice when the (un)timely Saturday evening call was received.

"My pup swallowed my daughter's pajamas." (She was a first grader.)

"Come over in about ten minutes," was my reply.

My quick injection of apomorphine (an emetic to induce vomiting) was followed by a two-minute hiatus and some pre-retching anxiety. Then with a huge belch, up came a slightly damaged, one-piece set of P.J.s, still intact.

The stomach contents were now interlaced with the pajama fabric, but the pup still had a hungry interest in these savory morsels. So I deposited the bundle in a trash can out near our heavily used incinerator.

When I, still a young doctor, told the staff members about the weekend escapade on the following Monday morning, no one really believed my story. Not to be discouraged by their skepticism, I took a rolled up newspaper, recovered the now significantly odorous nightwear, and presented it to them for inspection, much to their dismay. I may be accused at times of embellishment, but never exaggeration. I also learned that nylon tricot material becomes very slimy when wet, a condition compounded to the nth degree when combined with a Saint Bernard's saliva.

I have titled this tale of swallowed objects "The Revenge of the Retriever." It's my favorite.

It was a warm afternoon in August 1971 when my practice receptionist/secretary/technician/surgical assistant/kennel person received the call. My entire staff (she and I) confidently told the owner of "Jake," an eight-year-old lumbering black Labrador, that he could easily handle an adult dosage of an oral antihistamine for what appeared to be a nasty bee sting. Jake had been wandering through an apple orchard and had arrived home panting and upset with heavy swelling above the left eye, not unlike the goose egg you would expect from a Mike Tyson right hook.

Four hours later as I was preparing to leave for the night, my answering service relayed a new message to me from Jake's owners: he was now staggering around, bumping into things, panting, and appeared to be in great deal of pain. When Jake arrived at the hospital with his owners thirty minutes later, it was obvious that they had not exaggerated his condition. He also had a fever of 106 degrees.

With the able assistance of his young owners, I placed the dog in a cooling bath, catheterized the cephalic vein, and administered the time-honored medications for serious bee stings and high fevers — dipyrone and steroids. Jake's high temperature was very responsive to the treatment, never exceeding 103 degrees for the next four days. While he was hospitalized, though, Jake developed severe bloody diarrhea, was unable to see, and had showed poor coordination. He also exhibited the unLabrador-like trait of anorexia — yes, he wouldn't eat.

As the days passed in the hospital, Jake received symptomatic treatment and intravenous fluid support that contributed to gradual improvement. The swollen area around the orbit of his eye changed dramatically. An area of skin about the size of a quarter necrosed (died) and sloughed, exposing underlying connective tissue and muscle. That was a good thing. During his ordeal Jake's tail never lost its ability to fan a breeze. After all he was a Labrador!

Following four days of systemic support, Jake was able to return home to continue his recovery. However, two days later a call came to us from his owners.

"Yes, Jake's back to himself totally. Are you sitting down, Doc? Guess what Jake threw up completely intact? A three-and-a-half-foot long copperhead snake with a few canine lacerations!"

You can be sure that this news brought a quick review of a veterinary medical text on snake bites that described the clinical symptoms and behavior exhibited by Jake. Who would have thought of such a scenario?

I tried to imagine this curious black Lab watching the coiled reptile and then extending an inquisitive right paw to see if it would move and ZAP! OUCH! "Why that snake just bit me. I think I'll swallow it after a few good shakes."

If only I had x-rayed Jake's stomach on presentation. But when is the last time any veterinarian took an abdominal radiograph of a dog with a "bee sting" on its head?

Over the years I have learned a lot of life's lessons from the pets I have treated and the owners I have met. Things in life are not always what they seem. Innocent events can have serious outcomes; dangerous events can have positive resolutions. Making an effort to solve a problem is half the battle. Dedicated pet owners and caring veterinary practitioners are important allies because they both want the best life they can provide for the pets that give so much unconditional love. It is important to remember that good things happen when we lead from the heart and keep bad things out of our stomachs!

CHAPTER VIII

There Is No Love in Calories!

My personal experience has confirmed this truism: "My dog would rather eat at your house than mine."

"Why is that?" you ask. Because too many clients believe that if their pets are fat, they are happy.

Here are some classic comments from pet owners:

"Whenever my dad goes out for dinner, he asks the waitress to put aside a piece of his steak *before* she brings it out. This way he can't possibly forget his doggie bag. It would completely ruin dinner out if dad would come home without a treat for 'Fritz.'"

"She may not live as long, being as heavy as she is, but doesn't she look happy?"

"My husband and I share feeding responsibilities for our dog, and occasionally we discover that we've both fed him his dinner. Funny, our dog never tells us he's already eaten." (Now that's a Labrador owner for you!)

Frequently, I see someone, other than the owner, bring in a pet for an examination. Or sometimes a "nonfeeder" is present but the "feeder" stays way out of earshot during the visit. This used to puzzle me until I realized that the owners knew that my "overweight pet lecture" was imminent. Even though they knew I wouldn't "shoot the messenger," that didn't make my message any easier to take.

Far be it from me to miss an opportunity to orate on the health risks of obesity in pets. Hopefully, these clients take away an information morsel (a low-fat one for sure!) that would convince the canine chef at home to change his ways. Certainly, heavy dogs can live a long life, but normally weighted ones have a much better opportunity to do so. In the larger dog breeds, the most common reason for euthanasia is not kidney failure, cancer, or heart failure. Rather it is the loss of dignity that comes from an overweight body punishing the joints until mobility is severely compromised.

Every pet is at the mercy of an owner who defines love in terms of calories, and that pet often becomes an unwitting victim of good intentions. Most people don't want to hear advice on this subject and rarely consider it pertinent. I suppose it often hits too close to home, surfacing two issues instead of one.

In many situations the problem exists not only with "Rover" but also with the owners. Regardless of how well you know

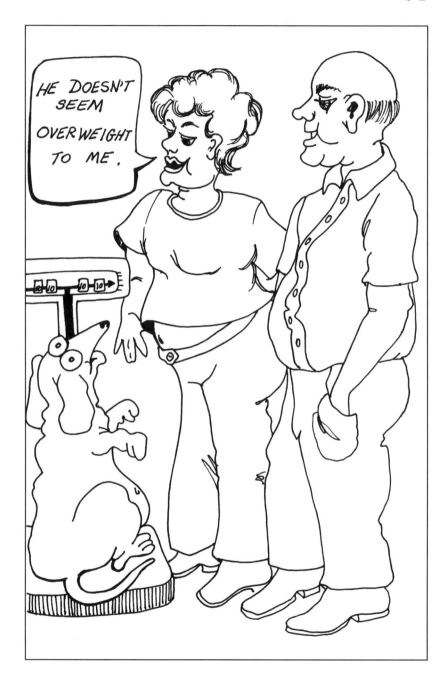

someone or how experienced a veterinarian might be dealing with sensitive subjects, it is difficult to broach the subject of overweight when either the mom or dad or both are on the heavy side. Unless they make light of their own figures first, I don't go there.

A study done in the United States during the early 1970s showed that 40 percent of owners who had fat canines were overweight themselves, and 40 percent of these people did not recognize that their pets were obese. In these homes, the pet is in major trouble from day one. The increasing cases of obesity in the U.S. today suggest that the situation for pets is likely to be at dangerous levels.

Fat begets fat, so if a veterinarian is fortunate enough to intervene with a pup or kitten early in their lives, there is hope. But once bad habits have gotten out of hand, it may be too late.

There are the two proven methods that help most to promote healthy eating habits and weight control in dogs because they help your pet put its "fork" down between mouthfuls: 1) feed dry, dry (no, I'm not stuttering!) food, and 2) split the daily feed ration into two meals.

The slower you eat, the less you eat because it satisfies the satiation (chewing) center in your brain. The same principle applies to your dog. By feeding twice a day, the dog is "starving" after only twelve hours instead of "really starving" after twenty-four hours. Two feedings may slow down the dog's sense of hunger urgency. Dry food fed this way may also foster an increased degree of mastication. Where there are multiple dogs in the house, this will also moderate the tendency for competitive eating, something we've had to manage in our two-Labrador household.

Early in my career I saw a dog swallow an entire sixteen-ounce can of dog food in one gulp, regurgitate the contents, and then with some attempt at chewing, inhale it again in what seemed to be in a split second.

This canine gourmand was a mixed black Lab, if memory serves me. At the time there was a brand of canned food whose consistency was solid (not unlike Spam). You had to open both ends of the can entirely and push out the contents — a three-inch diameter, six-inch long mass. I thought I was seeing things when I saw that dog inhale the whole blob. But later in my career, I was equally astounded when an English setter swallowed an entire, intact tennis ball. Dogs have some amazing "talents."

I was calling a client with the results of a thyroid function test on their laid-back, heavy, tail-wagging "Schmokie," a collie. I was hoping to find an abnormal test value so I could promote a healthier lifestyle and shinier coat for their longhaired pet.

The owners were a youngish couple, extremely fit themselves, who were well aware that an overweight collie was genetically prone to joint breakdown problems. Therefore, general health, especially in the later years of this breed, is a profoundly important issue. Since dogs have no vanity, we must promote a healthy level of vanity for them.

When the phone rang, Kathy answered and I responded, "Hello, I'm calling to. . ."

"Mark feeds him! I don't," she declared.

It was quite obvious that she recognized my voice. Kathy had pleaded innocence even before I could relate the "good news" about the bad test results.

I had no intention of blaming Kathy as Mark had already owned up to most of the calorie loading. Had Kathy come in with Mark for the visit, she might have been struck by my lecture on "the perils of pet obesity" and done more to promote a change in her husband's feeding patterns.

When I stop and ask a client how much they feed their dog, I'm not surprised anymore.

"We only feed eight cups of food a day and the bag says eight to eleven cups. We can't understand why our dog is gaining weight while we're underfeeding her?"

In the eyes of this owner, she was giving "Queenie" the proper amount of food.

If your seventy-five pound dog is on a treadmill twenty-three hours a day, you can feed what the pet food company recommends. Twenty-three hours is certainly an exaggeration, but the animals in a nutrition research lab are doing many hours of active exercise. At your house and ours, pets tend to rest and relax about twenty-three hours a day and exercise for one hour. And that's no exaggeration.

Weight gain is certainly more directly proportional to calories placed in the oral cavity than lack of exercise, much to the chagrin of many owners. Active exercise will burn up a few calories and help maintain muscle tone. The only way to keep on top of this tremendously important health matter is frequent weigh-ins. (That applies to people as well!)

There is a rather important second reason why the bag of pet food suggests eight to eleven cups per day. The more your pet eats, the more food you purchase. Unfortunately, for some pet food manufacturers, profit comes at the expense of your dog's waistline and despite your veterinarian's wrath.

Our dear friends had a cat named "Ashley" that lived well into her late teens in spite of a keen determination to eat and eat and eat. She was a heavy fourteen pounds in her early years, and with due diligence Don and Nan kept her near that weight for a full fourteen years.

I am an early riser and whenever we stayed with these friends, my trip down the steps in the morning was made quite adventurous by this ankle-rubbing, highly vociferous black feline. With lights off, the morning darkness blended with Ashley, making each step a test of my agility and athletic dexterity. (Luckily, I never fell.)

Ashley always led me without choice toward the kitchen cupboard that contained, you guessed it, her Cat Chow. I followed to a "T" the family directions that "x" number of pieces were to be counted and put before her at each regularly scheduled feeding. Believe me when I say, Ashley never let them skip a meal, let alone be late for one.

Not infrequently, these friends would stay with us for a weekend. Don was a crafty engineer (or so he thought) and upon leaving his home to come to ours, he would put out three bowls of the dry food for Ashley. These bowls were strategically placed around the house, actually hidden in a variety of locations. This ploy was designed so that Ashley would "save" some food for the following day.

Twenty minutes into a trip to visit us, Nan realized that they had forgotten their hanging clothes, so they decided to return home to retrieve them. They were greeted by Ashley wearing a Cheshire-cat face and all three bowls licked clean. They were outwitted by their cat, but if you ever had the chance to meet Don, well — no big surprise!

Another case of "food morsel counting" was a four-year-old golden retriever owned by a beautiful couple whom I've always had a kind feeling toward. "Yogi's" parents were both high school educators, and Mike was an extremely successful golf coach at a local high school. I suspect that a good part of the program's success was because he inherited good players. He certainly couldn't have produced that many, as I had seen him golf. In fact he was no better a golfer than I was and that isn't so good.

Their only "child" was their very loved dog, Yogi. Yogi's obesity was totally counter to the usual situation where the dog's physique mimics its owners. In this case, his "parents" were a vigorous, athletic couple. They had Yogi on a strict regimen of low fat, dry food and actually counted out each piece of food at each feeding.

True to all veterinary texts, the picture of the sleepy-faced golden with dull coat and a weight problem was indeed the classic profile of a hypothyroid dog. After four months of oral medication, his coat started to brighten and most importantly an eighteen-pound weight loss resulted. Yogi went from a large-bellied couch potato to a trim-waisted golfer's caddy.

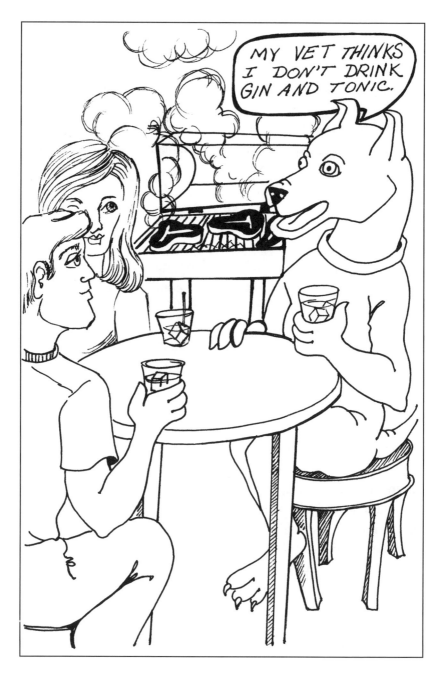

"Brandy" was a blond, overweight cocker spaniel who, over the nine years of his life, actually ended up enjoying (tolerating?) the attention he experienced during his visits to our practice. But this cocker, weighing a full sixty-three pounds, was truly overweight. Now sixty-three pounds on a tall dog is pretty easy to lift onto the exam table but a short-legged cocker is another story.

Part of the accumulated weight was due to the Thursday evening dinner ritual that he shared with his owners. Three, eight-ounce filet mignons were ordered weekly and delightfully grilled following a gin and tonic. Brandy was an integral part of this dinner with cocktails. I'm certain, however, that he never saw or tasted the Beefeaters gin, but I'm sure he enjoyed his weekly filet! I never could figure our why his "parents" never told me what time they fed him on Thursdays!

"Homeboy" was the overweight feline of an elderly spinster whom our entire staff came to know well because of her frequent taxi trips to our office. When her cat had to stay overnight for any reason, I would return him to Mildred on my way home from the practice.

As the years passed, Mildred had to move to an assisted-living facility, so Homeboy stayed with us. Every Tuesday evening, I would take Homeboy to visit her for a short period. Actually, I recall that I spent more time *getting* to her room than being *in* her room. Residents of these facilities thoroughly enjoy every visitor — *anybody's* visitors. This is true as much for the four-legged variety as it is for the two-legged, maybe more. Anyone who takes a pet into a retirement/nursing home knows full well that this is no exaggeration.

Weight was becoming a health hazard for Homeboy. The general health of the six-year-old feline was very important to Mildred, so we hospitalized him for two weeks to see what we could find. Blood work did not reveal any endocrinological cause for his obesity, so the staff started to portion out his food rations piece by piece and also invoke an exercise program. This consisted of running (well, at least forced rapid walking) him up and down a forty-foot long hallway.

Homeboy was, at the very least, a "C" cup as measured by the pendulous fat accumulation of his lower abdomen so commonly seen in cats of both sexes that are neutered. His "belly" would sway back and forth hitting the floor as he was plodded along on his health marches.

We learned two things from this two-week exercise program which turned out to be an exercise in frustration. First, his owner obviously had not been overfeeding him and second, our practice's "weight loss spa" was a failure! At best he lost a scant three ounces.

Shortly thereafter, Mildred fell and broke her hip. Her death followed not long afterwards. During her last weeks Homeboy and I visited the rehab center where she passed away. As "the boy" and I walked down the hallway, voices from "nowhere" would call out to us: "Are you here to see me?"

But we were there just to see Mildred. When we entered her room, there was no question in my mind that the delight on the face of our dear old friend was directed totally toward her long-time companion, her darling Homeboy. I don't know if she even remembered that I was there too. That didn't matter. Though her

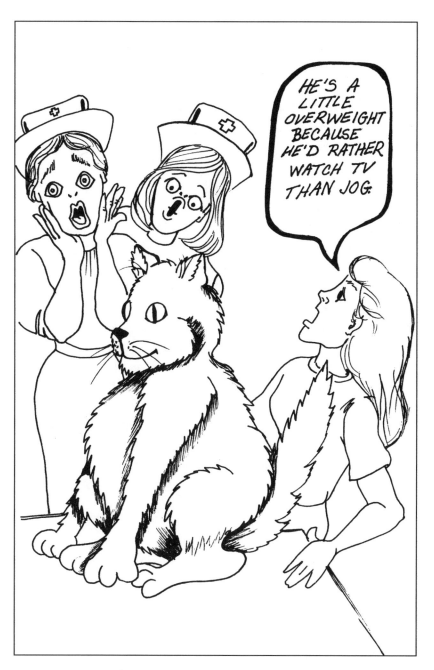

eyesight was failing, Homeboy's obesity made him much easier to see. I guess that is one positive side of being "large."

After Mildred's passing, Homeboy was adopted by one of our dedicated, senior employees, Dusty. She gave him a wonderful home for his later years. Although his weight never changed, his name did. She called him "Homefry."

There is great comfort in knowing that love is blind but that love still requires our special attention. True love, unconditional love, forgives our flaws and our bad days while it celebrates our existence and our achievements. The tail that wags with unbridled enthusiasm when we return from an outing and the loving family member or friend that hugs us when we seem down give us strength and courage when we need it. We don't need to be good-looking, smart, physically fit, or wealthy to deserve these reminders that we are loved. But we do need to remember just how fragile life can be — that those whom we need and who need us are merely mortal. Protecting our own health and the health of our pets becomes the most precious gift we give out of love. The next time you feel like giving your pet an extra helping, give it a warm hug instead.

CHAPTER IX

Tough Choices — Right Decisions

It was perhaps the only time in my life that I ever appreciated the smell of a cigarette.

This tale started during Easter week several years back when spring was in the air. Well, at least it was supposed to be. A very late winter storm had laid down nearly ten inches of snow.

A call came into our office that a dog's death was imminent followed by an urgent request, "Could someone stop by to euthanize a cancer-ridden, one-hundred-plus pound Saint Bernard?" This dog's home was not that far out of my way, so my offer to make a house call was readily accepted. The storm had abated and was replaced by high winds. Predictably, these winds led to heavy drifting, and I guessed correctly that this family did not own a snow shovel. These owners were oblivious to everything around them, so overwhelmed and consumed were they by the dire condition of their beloved pet.

So I plodded up their walk that had drifted shut, snow covering my shoes and knee-deep in some places. As the door opened, I was immediately overcome by the ammoniacal odor of stale urine and cigarette smoke, and I was not even in the house.

I knew my clothing would end up smelling like a stinging combination of nicotine and ammonia, both together being better than either alone. Certainly, my Labs would enjoy some olfactory research upon my arrival home when they would have a chance to check out my clothing like a pair of detectives.

Both owners greeted me graciously and thankfully as they puffed away on their cigarettes. "We knew we couldn't wait any longer," they said, "but we feel so badly doing it to him. We love him so much." (More on *this* viewpoint later.)

Their pet had been diagnosed with metastatic lung cancer. The primary site of the tumor was the spleen that had been removed late the previous year. The dog lay on a large, thick blanket under which was a sheet of plastic material. Unable to move, this large Saint Bernard had lain for four days in his own wastes. He had been kept as clean as possible, but all I could think of was how blind love can be.

My job this night was to deliver an intravenous, euthanizing drug that would humanely end this dog's suffering. The difficulty arose in this particular situation from several factors:

1. The dog was lying on the floor.
2. The light source was a handheld desk lamp.
3. My knees literally needed replacing.
4. A hanging veil of smoke affected visibility.
5. The condition of his veins was terrible.

Otherwise, no problem! The owners could not bear to watch the procedure, but at least they demonstrated some lamp-holding prowess.

This kind act — the final moment of a lifetime of love and care — takes less than fifteen seconds to perform under normal circumstances. The only discomfort is the prick of the needle as the drug itself is painless. The procedure is no different than our having a blood sample drawn at a local medical laboratory. I am embarrassed to say this, although I shouldn't be, but it took twenty-seven different needle sticks involving four different needles and a total of five veins to start the kind intravenous overdose of anesthesia.

This ailing dog had little blood pressure as he lay semicomatose on the blanket. This made the veins extremely difficult to locate by sight or feel, thus impeding administration of this drug of kindness. The owners had literally hoped their dog would die on his own over that weekend. Ironically, he had been scheduled for euthanasia the *previous* Friday, one week before Easter weekend. But the owners had canceled that appointment. Now, a once proud Saint — a mere shell of himself this day — continued to suffer, being kept alive well beyond his time. So many people just don't understand!

These owners had not followed my most important caregiver's credo: make the decision to euthanize the day *before* it must be done. People use guilt as the reason they wait for their pets to die which, with cats and dogs, happens statistically only 5 to 8 percent of the time. Left on their own, animals don't/can't pick a time to die with dignity and minimal suffering. People let their hearts rule their heads and do not take advantage of a wonderful opportunity to alleviate suffering and protect their pets' quality of life.

Yes, all of this started on Good Friday and ended on Easter Monday. Uncharacteristically, I was still extremely angry with these owners for their poor and delayed decision-making. I found it difficult to be supportive of them at that moment, and I know I avoided eye contact as we shook hands goodbye. That was a fairly long time ago, and as much as I don't like to admit it, I know that I wouldn't feel any differently today.

I have lain flat on my stomach in someone's living room to euthanize a six-pound Yorkie. I've put down a Hollywood shag dog on my hands and knees having forgotten my glasses. In both these instances some angel on my shoulder guided the needle and all went smoothly. For this I am thankful, because there is nothing worse than a missed vein and unexpected pet whimpering when the owners are already feeling remorseful about the moment and maybe — though unnecessarily — some guilt.

For years Pete and Liz have been two of my favorites even though we don't agree on her favorite radio show — a political call-in program. It came time to do the right and kind act for their wonderful Airedale terrier, "Reggie." Pete had dug a grave next to their house in an area of beautiful plantings. This was a willing house call, as Reggie had earned everyone's love, including mine.

The three of us knelt on an old quilt in the afternoon sunlight and said our goodbyes to Reggie as he fell into an endless sleep. An expected moment of silence followed and then hugs and words about faithfulness, giving more than he received, and other tributes.

I then participated in the funeral by taking Liz's position as a pallbearer, helping Pete to wrap Reggie in his quilt and carry him graveside. The burial site was on the opposite side of the house so we proceeded to that area. I was astonished to see a rectangular grave about five feet long and two feet wide. When Pete jumped into the grave, I thought he would disappear completely. As it turned out, he was only waist deep as we placed this finest of Airedales in his final resting place.

Pete then leaped athletically out of the grave, returning my smile with one of his own. It was a sad occasion made joyful by this engineer's hole dug with magnitude and precision. Early on, Pete had asked my advice on the depth of the grave, and in my experience I suggested that three feet was plenty deep.

Of course, Pete just had to be as close to perfection as possible. By then our tears had become smiles and the moment was one to remember. As I returned to my car past the rear of their house, I heard a noise and recognized that radio show playing through Liz's open kitchen window.

Never to be forgotten was the time a geriatric toy poodle had reached its maximum years of quality life. His senior mother was most appreciative of my offer to bury him with all my personal pets in our vegetable garden.

All went smoothly, that is, until the very next day when a knock on our back door was, you guessed it, the poodle's owner.

"I've decided to bury him on a friend's farm," she declared. What's the saying, "I'm a day late and a dollar short?"

"Pierre" was already in the ground. Fortunately, his interment included a pillowcase coffin, so he was expeditiously exhumed and placed in the cardboard box his "mother" now provided.

I really never believed her story of why she wanted him out of my yard. She certainly had trusted me while he was alive, why not when he was dead? In all, I was thankful that I had buried Pierre in that pillowcase and that I had not dug a grave like Reggie's!

A longhaired, black mixed retriever-type dog had been a patient with us for years. The family's children completed college and were into the early stages of married life. Of course, this longtime canine friend needed and deserved a kind ending and a proper burial. Early kidney failure had added to the woes of this severely arthritic dog.

This was a house call to remember. As I walked up the driveway to reach the front door, I heard a voice calling from the backyard over the fence.

"We're back here" was the instruction. And I do mean *we*. A total of nine were gathered, if memory serves me, including several grandchildren, daughters, sons-in-laws, and mother.

They all chose to be present at this solemn moment after I described what would take place. A semicircle was formed as we congregated at graveside. Remember now, I said this was a longhaired dog. Now you must appreciate that an audience adds to my hopes and prayers that all goes smoothly. Okay, it creates increased pressure, too.

As it turned out there was no electricity at the grave site. I needed to use my clippers to shave the leg and make a vein accessible. Consequently, the family entourage and I (ten in all) along with "Onyx" walked in file up to their deck where there was an electrical outlet. Shaving accomplished, we returned to our original site and all went smoothly. Looking back, in a lighter vein, the only thing missing in this cortege was a horse-drawn casket.

Around the holiday season, specifically Thanksgiving through New Year's day, many pets are euthanized. There are several reasons for this and most all are good ones. Certainly veterinarians would never imply that people just say "it's time; let's do it," and move on. And for sure, I am not suggesting that people elect to euthanize old or ailing pets to avoid any inconvenience or disruption while they are focused on the festivities of the holiday. Although a fair number of people worry that the timing of their decision may look like that is the reason. This concern is no reason to defer doing the right thing.

There are very legitimate factors that move these important decisions along during the holidays. As winter moves ever nearer in mid-November, our thoughts go to the fourteen-year-old cocker spaniel who must drag itself outside into the wintry blasts or to the equally loved English setter who faces the cold season in his outside kennel awaiting next September's small game season. Or how about the chubby, elderly pug that can no longer walk the icy surroundings with its ungainly elderly master? So seasonally we foresee these patterns of potential struggle and decision making.

When children are away at college, only the parents witness the rapid decline of their pets on a daily basis. So before these final decisions are made they conclude, "Let's wait until the children get home when we can all say our goodbyes." Often these young adults have the duty to take these pets to a veterinarian's office for their final visit. Their parents just can't bring themselves to do it, even though it is the right thing to do. Again I repeat that this decision should be made the day before euthanasia *has* to be done. The holidays are a time of family joy and celebration and to have a failing geriatric pet not enjoying the camaraderie is fair to no one.

We must think quality of life for our pets and not the quantity of years. Time and again we see pets actually waiting until a daughter or son comes home from school and then that pet tells them, "It's time." When people feel guilty about a decision that takes the life of a "good friend," they need support to assure them that their decision — made on the animal's behalf — is done with the head and not the heart. Selfish owners keep their pets alive because they find it difficult to let go, so those animals suffer in the name of quantity and not quality of life.

A poodle-owning client became extremely distraught when her pet died before we could spay it for an infected uterus the following morning. This dehydrated failing older poodle had an intravenous drip in her overnight that, hopefully, would have rendered the needed surgery somewhat safer. But we never got that far.

The strangeness of this situation started with the owner gaining access to our hospital's interior unbeknownst to any staff members. Shortly afterward, she was discovered there with her

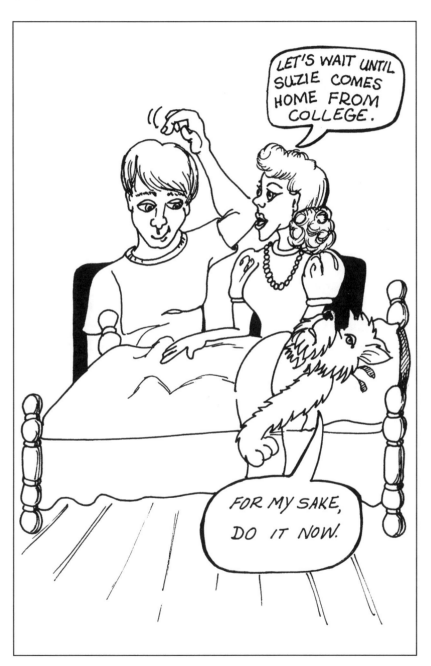

dog, "Monique," that had died. (It was surmised the woman had hidden in the hospital overnight.)

This client proceeded to blame everyone on our staff for deliberately killing her beloved dog. She became unbalanced, carrying the dog's body through our waiting room and calling us a murderous bunch of doctors, screaming as loud as possible.

Now this tale really takes a peculiar turn. In a section of our local newspaper two days later, the headline read: "Woman attempts burial at local cemetery." The article went on to say that a woman acting strangely was seen walking among the headstones carrying an infant casket. She also had a folded up travel shovel in her possession.

An observant neighbor called the police, and they apprehended her quickly. Jumping to conclusions, the officers assumed she was trying to bury a baby. But this ranting and raving woman was attempting to bury her pet.

Subsequently, a police examination of the casket proved her claim. She ultimately paid a fine for trespassing. All were relieved that there was no foul play concerning a newborn. I know she forever thought foul play on our part caused the loss of her Monique, and I'm certain she pleaded her case to the police. In all, this was a very sad case.

"Katie," a mixed terrier one month short of her seventeenth year, was brought to our office. She was in total collapse, obviously ready for the great gift of love and kindness — euthanasia.

As her loving caregivers, the Webbs, and I stood there, I realized that they were providing as much comfort and support

to me as I was to them. Shared sadness soon turned to a celebration of her life.

"Do you remember the time she vocally challenged a
Chesapeake Bay retriever in the waiting room when she was just
a four-pounder?"

More memories followed. How glad I was to have been
there for them and them for me as they held Katie in their arms.

Mrs. Webb then declared, "We've loved her so much that we
can't go through this again. She'll be our last one."

I quickly reminded her that this was the third time over
many years that she said the same words. I know that, in time, I
will see the Webbs again with a new "friend!"

The greatest test of love is the test of courage. Making the
right decisions in difficult situations for the good of those we
love is the measure of the true love we proclaim. From the
beginning of life, our pets depend on us. Throughout their lives
we teach them that their unconditional love and loyalty are
rewarded by our dedication to their care, training, and protection. They trust us to watch over them, make decisions for them,
and to love them. They depend on us for a good life as they grow
and thrive; they also depend on us to keep them from pain, suffering, and loss of viability. When they are unable to be there for
us, we need to be there for them. Giving them rest and freedom
from decline when they "tell" us that they can no longer live a
quality life is our duty. When it's your turn to make your first or
yet another tough choice, always know that it is a right decision,
made out of your love and courage.

CHAPTER X

The Home Front

Every day for more than four decades in practice, I see the warmth and uniqueness of family units that include a special connection between people and pets — all kinds, all shapes, all sizes, all ages and types. This is something special that I share with my clients and with my own family.

My wife, two daughters, and I have experienced all the joys and sorrows that living with pets can bring — our "animal children" have been Labrador retrievers, one West Highland white terrier, and cats of several varieties. They have filled our lives with memorable moments, which make us part of a very wonderful animal-loving community. Here are some personal moments that have been commemorated in one-of-a-kind ways by certain four-legged friends — the good, the bad, and the ugly!

I met Joan, my wife of forty years, in the most romantic of fashions — as the result of a feline castration. My in-laws-to-be had brought in their black cat for neutering.

It was 1960 and I was a second-year graduate student at the University of Pennsylvania Veterinary School. Every Wednesday evening I manned the office of a suburban practitioner. Answering phones, cleaning up, and discharging hospitalized pets were my forte.

A December snowstorm occurred that fateful Wednesday. The phone rang about 7 PM and the young female voice on the line asked, "Are you the student?"

"Yes," I answered. "How may I help you?"

It was Joan eager to pick up the family cat, "Jasper," but her father had not yet come home from work with their only car. Being the helpful fellow and gentleman that I was — and still am — I offered to give her and Jasper a ride home if she could get to the animal hospital. To this day, Joan's mother cannot believe she took a cab to the animal hospital to retrieve that cat.

Four hours later at 11 PM, I was still at Joan's home when the phone rang. It was my worried mother. It seems that my parents had called the veterinary office and my boss to inquire about my whereabouts. The doctor had no idea where I was but checked the discharge files, and from my punch-out time, he deduced that I must have taken a client and patient home. Joan and I saw each other for eleven consecutive nights while she was home on Christmas break from college.

Our relationship blossomed early that first evening as we
pulled in at her house. As she walked down the icy driveway,
clutching Jasper, she fell on her plaid-covered buttocks.
Automatically I asked, "Is your cat okay?" She really *fell* for me
then and there! We were married two years later.

We were in our new house only two weeks and a long anticipated trip to *Europe on $5.00 A Day* awaited us. (And as this
popular book title challenged, we came mighty close to accom-
plishing that feat. But the year *was* 1967.) My in-laws were to
drive us to Kennedy Airport, and on the way we would drop off
our Lab, "Midnight," at the animal hospital where I was
employed.

As we readied for our departure almost on schedule, we discovered, much to our chagrin, that Midnight had disappeared.
Because we had been in this house for only two weeks and
because we were located on a busy highway, our concern for our
very first retriever was clearly justified. As we started our
search, negative thoughts dominated.

We trudged through the surrounding unharvested cornfields
and some interspersed tree lines. We whistled and called — all
to no avail. I crossed the highway, hoping my worst fears were
unfounded. I ran through the dried, upright corn stalks oblivious
to a wasp nest on my right. As I exited the rows, I realized a few
wasps were starting to pay me back for disturbing their abode.

Our search ended in a neighbor's driveway bordering the
cornfield. As I was about to knock on their door to leave a
description, I heard a subtle whining from his open garage.
There she was — scared to death but full of joy. And those were

the two feelings we shared also, along with a great sense of relief. Midnight seemed no worse for the wear although we'll never know what she experienced that afternoon.

Predictably, I never felt the pain of those wasp stings until we left for New York. The beautiful vacation reminiscences will always be tempered by my memories of the soreness and swelling in the crook of my elbow and behind my knee on that six-hour flight to Munich. I guess a wasp's gotta do what it's gotta do!

In 1967 I was just four years out of the University of Pennsylvania Veterinary School and very impressionable, but always candid. So when I got this message, "My Westie needs a C-section. I'm an OB-GYN and I went to Princeton," I immediately took the call.

For over thirty-five years Alan and I and our families have remained friends. He ably assisted in his bitch's Caesarian, and a mutual respect developed immediately. When one of the pup's eyes had not opened by the time it was ten days old, he and I did a quick and easy, lid-splitting procedure. Her left eye was fine but her right eye was not identifiable. All that was there was clotted blood with a raisin-like eyeball. A few weeks later, an enucleation (eye removal) was performed, and shortly thereafter this sweet Westie pup became part of *our* family.

Her facial hair had been shaved as a result of the surgery. But when it grew back, no one could tell she was one eye short. So "Twinkle" joined our two black Labs.

Several years later, our three canines would spend Monday evenings in an outside 20 x 20 foot pen at our home — a pen that sported an elegant doghouse for their use in bad weather. In those days, Joan spent three hours on Monday nights as my receptionist. When we would return home each Monday to our three dogs, we would release them from the pen, and Twinkle would run the forty yards to our house while the two Labs ran up to the barn to chase the pigeons. Well, this went on for months when we noticed that Midnight was going with the Westie instead of with "Jemima."

At the time we thought nothing of this. Then on one of those nights, Midnight ran into the lamp post near the back porch. Again, nothing seemed amiss to us until shortly thereafter. As she leaped onto our raised patio, she whacked her forelegs on the eighteen-inch high wall. Suddenly we realized we had a blind dog. Midnight had gone blind over a long period of time (progressive retinal atrophy) and had acclimated so well to her surroundings that we didn't notice.

So we ended up with a one-eyed dog, a normally-sighted dog, and one that was "ophthalmologically challenged." And you know what? Until our young twins started leaving large items out of their normal positions, we couldn't see any difference among our dogs — a least not without an eye chart.

A year after moving into our house, one of our house cats disappeared for eighteen days. We had written "Jacob" off with the sadness that clouds the issue when there's really no closure.

On the eighteenth day post-disappearance we were scheduled to leave on a week's vacation. We sat on our front porch discussing whatever and heard a rustling in the ground cover in the shrubs. Careful exploration of the pachysandra revealed the recently returned prodigal cat.

In spite of having lost several pounds, this bedraggled black feline was purring away. Had he returned only one day later, we just know he would have died out there. Where he had been and what he had been through we'd never know, but the simple joy of Jacob's return knew no limits.

The year 1969 was an important one for our growing family. We opened the doors of Lehigh Valley Animal Hospital on July 20, beginning a thirty year adventure in veterinary practice ownership. To help us celebrate this momentous occasion, our country landed a manned spacecraft on the moon. We felt quite honored!

Just two months prior to this, Jemima whelped thirteen Labrador pups, eight of which were yellow and the remainder black. We have beautiful, old slides of these rascals sharing three bowls of puppy chow. Not to be outdone, our well-bred Siamese queened six kittens that September.

Wow. Two large litters! However wonderful these two events were, they just couldn't compare with the moment Joan delivered the third litter of the year. Two full-term, fraternal twin daughters emerged on November 22, 1969, and came home to stay that Thanksgiving Day. How appropriate.

Rarely do small animal practitioners witness a solo birth and that remained a truism for me in 1969.

We didn't realize how much we talked to our pets until our children came along.

Our daughters were born six years after our marriage. Our two Labs responded to the kind and gentle words we directed at our infants. Thinking, as always, that they were the objects of our exaggerated and affectionate tones, their trim canine bodies were often poised to join the four of us on the sofa — always forbidden territory.

Our three cats, one of which was Siamese, deemed the newborns beneath their dignity and treated them with amusing disdain but growing curiosity as days turned into months. They came to realize that their new "siblings" were here to stay. The only trouble was that a Siamese cry for attention often sounded like an infant in distress. But we adapted and were always happier to run up the stairs to pick up a whining feline than a crying child.

Before our daughters reached kindergarten age, we would rent a place at the beach very reasonably for two weeks in September after the vacation season ended. I would drive the four of us to the New Jersey shore, spend five days there, return home, spend four days at the practice, and then return to the beach to bring everyone home.

In the early 1970s, I couldn't justify two weeks away from my active solo practice. And that became a godsend. It seems one of our four-year-old daughters had gone back into her bedroom to retrieve some forgotten item from her closet before we left.

When I returned home five days later, it was quickly obvious that a cat was missing. While searching I heard some scratching sounds from the closet in the girls' room. When I slid the door open, out strolled the happiest, purringest cat you ever saw, probably wondering what he had done wrong to deserve solitary confinement for five days.

The only damage was, as you might expect, some urine and a BM on some folded sheets in a clothes basket. Neither cat nor linens were any worse for the wear. It would have been a different story had I stayed at the shore for the entire two weeks. As a veterinarian I don't recommend locking your cat in the closet when you go on vacation!

On New Year's Day 1984 I was on call for our practice when the answering service called to see if we had information about a missing Lab. They gave me a rabies tag number, which the veterinary assistant looked up and said, "Hey, that's one of your dogs!"

I called home and my surprised wife said that both Labs were in the backyard. Well, she was half right. "Dinah" had wandered into the new development where we would routinely power-walk our pair. Fortunately, Dinah had been taken in by a local home owner.

After a call and within fifteen minutes, Joan arrived to pick up the "errant child," and much to her embarrassment, Dinah took one look at her and headed for the rug under her "host's" dining room table. It seems her newly found "godparents" had been plying her with pretzels and potato chips while watching Joe Paterno's Penn State football team beating up on Bear Bryant's Crimson Tide, if memory serves me. As the reunited pair got ready to leave, the neighbor asked carefully, "She is your dog, isn't she?"

"Of course," Joan replied somewhat embarrassed.

This experience was a wake-up call for us. As it turned out, Dinah was in the early stages of what is now termed, cognitive dysfunction syndrome, a form of canine dementia.

Another of Dinah's solo jaunts also tested our nerves.

One night at bedtime, we let Dinah out for her pre-bed exercise. When she didn't respond to my calls, we knew something was amiss. I should add that the wind was howling with pouring rain blowing almost horizontally.

We searched the neighboring four acres of heavy woodland (now a shopping mall) both on foot and by directing the car's headlights into the trees. It was a fruitless search in the dark and bad weather. We feared the worst — that she had gotten her collar snagged somehow. We returned to our beds but slept very little while waiting for the early morning light.

At 6 AM the phone rang and our prayers were answered. Town houses were being built adjacent to and north of our property, and two new occupants had heard a whimpering dog around midnight. They discovered a black Lab that had fallen into recently dug footings and, because of the rain, could not extricate herself from her slippery dilemma.

My two-minute trip to the site revealed our muddied Dinah wrapped in a blanket and being hugged by two special people. Later that afternoon, I delivered our newly crowned knights in shining armor a bottle of wine that was small reward for what they had done. Believe me when I say it was offered with a great sense of both thanks and relief. After that episode Dinah was never allowed outside unsupervised.

Prior to the emergence of this new construction, our dogs never wandered to the north edge of our lot. We later learned that workmen next door would routinely share portions of their lunch boxes with them. What would you expect from a Labrador — the most food-driven breed ever created.

In June of 1984 one of our daughters was home alone as mother had taken her sister to a piano lesson. They were fourteen at the time. I received a call from the Pennsylvania State Police that they were investigating a break-in at our house some thirteen miles from where I was completing a cat spay. I didn't overreact or risk dropping the ovarian pedicle, but after one of our staff reported a constant busy signal after repeatedly dialing our home, my concerns came to the surface.

Fortunately, there were no injuries to child or pets, but the situation was very upsetting and disappointing. This event made for a very disturbing drama.

Normally, when the kids were home alone in their early teens, the two Labs were in the house with them. But today they were sunning themselves on the screened-in back porch. Alissa heard an abrupt, assertive knock on the front door and ran upstairs, peered out the window, and saw three strangely attired people — two men and a woman.

The dogs started to bark as our attempted burglars-to-be quickly walked to the side of the house. My daughter dialed a neighbor (there was no 911 back then) who in turn alerted the State Police who patrolled our township in the absence of a community police department.

By this time, Alissa had heard a thud from our kitchen, which was later determined to be a TV set which had been knocked off a window sill as one of the three intruders attempted a forced entry. A few steps farther and they were confronted by two fiercely barking, protective guardians of the manor — their tails wagging at a furious rate. "Come in and give us a hug in return for a big, wet lick," they begged.

The trio advanced through the porch door and were faced with the heavily bolted back door of our farmhouse, not to mention the continuing "inconvenience" of the canine sentries. A female State Trooper arrived on the scene just in time to see the disappointed threesome leave the property and jump into their vehicle. They were apprehended in short order after a brief chase on a major thruway.

When the court hearing took place some months later, both our family and the State Police were aghast when the judge bought the story that these intruders were merely looking for a used car dealership!

Their plea of not guilty was sustained in spite of testimony by our daughter and the trooper as well as hard evidence including a storm window with a palm print and a record of footprints in the ground cover beneath the window.

Needless to say, a letter to the editor from us regarding our criminal justice system and one to the judge from the county prosecutor did little except to satisfy our frustration and dismay.

Now if the Labs could have testified, I'm certain their input would have caused the judge to be fully convinced of the obvious motives of the defendants. We all realize that if the dogs had been in the house aggressively barking — with wagging tails unseen — those people would have been off the property posthaste. Damn those tails!

Who videotapes the TV shows in your house? Well, in my house my wife does. Admittedly, I've done it a few times but have had fewer successes than failures. The following event will serve as proof of my shortcomings around electronics.

It was time for our Labrador to make her film debut. When our older (by five minutes) daughter was a senior in high school, an English course required her to team up with a classmate and complete an audiovisual project. The two wrote a lengthy script after several hours of joyful collaboration. The production would star "Bess," our then five-year-old Lab, and our daughters' 1983 lime green Oldsmobile — lovingly christened "the Lime-o-sine." It was a senior citizen of a car, but as parents, we deemed this tank-like vehicle imminently safe for our girls.

A portion of the taped English project showed Bess at the steering wheel clad in a scarf, sunglasses, and topped with a baseball hat. It was a classic (at least by veterinary standards) and did them proud in class. They received the well-deserved grade of "A."

The following week my wife was out shopping, and I just had to tape the finals of some tennis tournament. You guessed it. I taped a valueless tennis match over a true family heirloom, now lost forever and irreplaceable. At least my "F" came *after* their "A."

"Annie," our Burmese cat, had a distinguished traveling career. She was flown in from Pittsburgh as a kitten and subsequently flew back twice for breeding. Shortly after her arrival in February 1988, we had to leave for an overnight to a human-only bed and breakfast. Not wanting to leave Annie home and

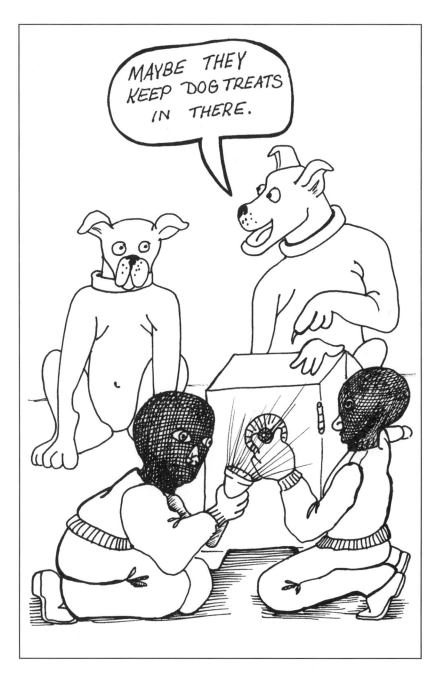

knowing about the "unwelcome mat" at the lodge, we were in a quandary, albeit short-lived.

Two suitcases for two people is very ordinary traveling fare. In those days, no one would ever question the contents. As it turned out, Annie loved our cat carrier disguised to look exactly like our very own luggage. Okay, it wasn't a cat carrier but really our converted suitcase. Because we were afraid to leave her alone in the room, she went with us to the tennis courts, the golf ball driving range, and the like.

Throughout her life, when any luggage appeared, Annie and her daughter "Bonnie" were right there helping to pack, leaping in and out joyfully. Of course, Annie's flights to western Pennsylvania for breeding were made in an official flying carrier. And whenever she saw that piece of equipment, she was *really* raring to go!

As a student for eight years in Philadelphia, our younger twin, Debbie, would occasionally have the opportunity to travel north an hour and a half by bus for an overnight at home. I would drive fifteen minutes to the bus depot and await her arrival. A huge hug and kiss followed as she leaped up with arms around my neck.

As we drove the short trip home, she would reflect and reminisce as she witnessed the slightest changes in her old neighborhood. The driveway to our house went along the north side of the barn, then made a quick left, and we were home. By this time our Labs sensed her arrival and were wagging their tails exuberantly to welcome her. She immediately dropped all her traveling possessions onto the black top and lay down in the grass.

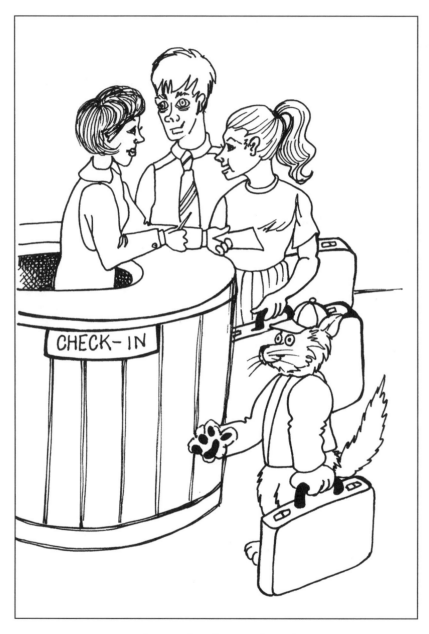

Room for three, please

She happily succumbed to the canine licks and hugs. Her mom, witnessing the arrival of the prodigal daughter from the doorway stood silent momentarily to enjoy the canine welcoming committee. Then with a feigned forlorn facial expression came the whiney, "Hi, I'm your mom. Remember me?"

Debbie's next seven years took her to Cincinnati for a residency and fellowship in pediatric otolaryngology (ear, nose, and throat), so visits were few and far between. "Why don't you both come out to visit as I've never had a chance to give you a tour of the hospital here!"

With jubilation Joan (as usual) made all the arrangements for the two-hour flight. She informed our daughter about the pending trip with much excitement. Then came a pregnant pause, and then, "Oh, could you bring 'Sara' along?" — our then two-year-old Lab.

"Of course, Honey, no problem" was the answer. That two-hour flight was replaced by a ten-and-a-half-hour drive. Fortunately, a canine-friendly motel was easily arranged both westbound and eastbound. The love between daughters and Labs over the years has given us untold joy.

In 1995 we introduced our then ten-week-old black Lab pup, "Sara" to our then seven- and five-year-old Burmese cats. It took about six to eight months for total acceptance by the older of the feline pair. Still today, although the younger feline tolerates Sara, full acceptance was never quite attained.

In March 1999, Julie, one of our techs, discovered a lump in Sara the exact size and firmness of the tip of your little finger. The growth was under the skin but near the muscle layer of her left rear leg in her upper thigh. The surgical excision was easily done.

The report from the pathologist surprised, stunned, frightened, and, in general, bewildered us. It described a highly malignant form of cancer. Specifically, the diagnosis was a grade III mast cell tumor. This finding was so rare that we sent the slides to a second veterinary school that corroborated the findings of the first. This is the worst form of this type of cancer, and only five percent of dogs live four years with it.

When we told our wonderful breeder our bad news, she insisted on giving us a gorgeous fourteen-month-old Lab that she had been showing to help us deal with our fears and trepidations. The new dog might offer us an emotional safety net should we lose Sara.

Within hours of "Sophie's" arrival Sara was literally forcing her stuffed animals into her new housemate's face, and Sophie loved every minute of it. Because the new dog was past that pushy puppy stage, she carried herself like a lady with maturity; she was also within ten pounds of the adult, Sara. Fortunately, our cats became tolerant fairly quickly too.

Sara underwent four further surgeries and a seven-week course of chemotherapy. One of the procedures was performed by a board-certified veterinary surgeon who removed a section of skin along with underlying tissues that measured 10½ x 5½ inches.

This was a difficult time for Sara and for us as we braced ourselves for the worst. We saw Sophie as our emotional insurance policy if Sara's life were to be shortened by her cancer. We hoped the void that Sara would leave would not be as hard to bear with another Lab already in our midst.

But as we all know, insurance policies always cost something. There's always the bottom line. And ours was the fact that

Sophie was being asked to acclimate to a family environment, a stark contrast to the kennel life and show dog atmosphere she had been raised in. So she arrived full of boundless energy. Every time we turned around, one of us was scolding her for bugging Sara mercilessly.

The sad part was that Sara mistook our constant reprimands — our stern voice inflections — to be directed toward her. So she responded in kind by going to her bed like a child with hurt feelings. Needless to say, no family member was happy at this point except for our newest member.

Enter Al and Lois. These wonderful people are parents of Betty, one of our most loyal and dedicated employees of over twenty-seven years. Coincidentally, their own Labrador retriever had recently been lost to cancer. A timely phone call and a trip to Pittsburgh resulted in the perfect home for Sophie — a place where she leads a true life of leisure with these friends. Since we have family in that city, we are able to take advantage of our "visiting privileges." Sophie keeps in touch with Sara through her annual Christmas card. This is truly a happily-ever-after story on all fronts since presently Sara's condition remains asymptomatic, five years after her diagnosis. Truly amazing.

In addition to my shared pet experiences as a veterinarian practice owner, husband, friend, and father, I have had some personal experiences that have marked me positively, and at times not so positively, throughout my life. These are things that I can only fairly attribute to my own peculiarities, my occasional flair for adventure, my periodic naiveté, my personal sense of duty, and my occasional tendencies to rush in where fools fear to tread. At the very least, some of these confessions are likely to take the gild off this veterinary lily.

In 1956 when I was a freshman in undergraduate school, an anatomy project was assigned as a second semester project. Three of us who were biology-chemistry dual majors (and all pledging the same fraternity) went to the professor to receive permission to do a joint project. We would construct a dog skeleton.

Joe's Uncle Steve was a Pennsylvania State Trooper who had access to roadkill. In short order we received the anticipated call, and the "body" was delivered to our campus. We named her "Belle."

Our first task was to convert Belle to her skeletal state. We had reasoned that there were two possible approaches to produce shiny, white bones: soaking her in brine (salt water) or burial unprotected in the earth. Because burial would not allow us to follow closely the transformational progress, we chose soaking.

First, we removed as much tissue as possible down to the bones. As you might expect, we did our collegiate best, but there still remained some soft tissue structures — specifically, the entire central nervous system (brain and spinal cord) within the skeleton itself. Also, we wanted to maintain the integrity of the four paws so all the support structures (ligaments and joint capsules) stayed with Belle temporarily. We found a steel drum, filled it with heavily salted water, and placed Belle carefully into it.

We placed the soaking Belle onto the second floor fire escape outside the laboratory of Steele Hall at Susquehanna University. Then we calmly went about college life as it should be: study, study, and more study followed by short breaks from studying for sports and dating.

Several months passed by and as winter melted into spring, the weekly drum checks showed little, if any, progress. Unfortunately, we failed to realize that the salt solution (the brine) was serving to preserve Belle's remains rather than allowing bacterial decomposition to take place.

So we formulated a "brilliant" plan to speed up the process. We would sneak into the lab after the end of Saturday morning classes and boil down the skeleton into beautiful ivory-like bones. I hope you never have the opportunity to smell the odor of boiling rotting flesh. It was only one of two times in my life that I wished I smoked. None of us did.

After that weekend, classes in the entire biology department were canceled for two days. Why we weren't dismissed from school is beyond me. The three of us were all good students, and our advisor probably deemed us worthy to remain. Or just maybe *he* was writing a book and needed some "dumb student" stories.

Fortunately, we did finally retrieve all three hundred plus bones and received a complete for our work, such as it was. My dad had made a wooden platform for Belle to honor her for her outstanding contribution to science. Most of her was standing but still to be attached were the tiny bones of the wrists, ankles, and paws. And they *were* tiny.

I was responsible to return the next fall semester with the totally completed project in hand. For whatever reason the skeleton never made it back to school but instead remained in my parent's basement for over twenty-five years. Sadly, the "Belle of the Ball" never graced Steele Hall.

"Extraordinary Dogs" is a wonderful two-hour documentary that describes how surprisingly amazing canines are. My neighbor and friend, who is president and general manager of our local PBS station, asked me to co-host a three hour segment during the station's pledge week. (Each featured segment of a particular show would be run and then followed by a discussion with on-screen commentators.) So it made sense for me to comment on this program from my perspective as a veterinarian.

One of the "pet" subjects we discussed during our on-air time was my strong opinion that chocolate Labs are more active and somewhat more hyper than their yellow and black counterparts. This is a view shared by many in the veterinary profession. I've always believed that there was Chesapeake Bay retriever blood in the chocolate Lab lineage that could account for the personality difference.

As you might imagine, the TV channel received an angry call from a local "chocolate" breeder. In no uncertain terms, I was admonished for my "know-it-all but know-nothing" statements. I took the time to "discuss" my viewpoint with her while another segment of "Extraordinary Dogs" was playing. However, she was not satisfied. As it turned out, my impact on public contributions during that pledge week was not particularly significant, so I was never invited back. That was fine with me.

A few years ago, I was asked by the pastor of the Central Moravian Church to make comments at the annual Blessing of the Animals outdoor service. I considered myself a real veteran of this calling because twelve years prior I had spoken at an

Episcopal service for St. Francis Day — St. Francis being the patron saint of animals.

Facing the Moravian congregation, I opened by saying, "My delivery this morning will not be what you are accustomed to at your services."

Their minister quickly retorted, "and I can't spay a cat as well as you can." The warm laughter from his church family immediately made me feel welcome.

My morning with the Moravians was tame compared to my earlier attempt at the pulpit in the Episcopal Church. The priest, a devout and elegant woman, had asked me to deliver a few words to recognize the importance of animals in our lives. I stood next to her as she introduced me to the congregation.

Church members, those seated in the pews and in the choir, had brought along their furry companions. The plan was to have these "Christian" pets parade down the aisle to the communion rail where she would bless them. My job was to deliver my well-written, overly-practiced two minutes of brilliant, yet worldly, wisdom. I had a sense, though, that trouble was brewing behind me in the choir loft. How right I was!

A handsome, large red feline had escaped its chorister-owner as I was speaking. As a result, that big ole cat was joyously meandering throughout the choir stalls, exploring the ankles, handbags, and shoe leather of the choir members. And there I was being completely upstaged by that blessed (or was it blasted) feline.

Clearly, I had lost my audience, and I don't remember anything whatsoever about my homily. But I do recall my wife making two important points — my Snoopy tie really looked good and I was not to quit my day job. There would be no seminary calling in my future either.

During the 1990s, I made many visits to a local nursing home to visit my parents. During one of those visits a bit of commotion arose in the hallway. It was caused by the annual Halloween visit of a group that truly excited the residents — Therapy Dogs in full costume!

The first to enter the room was "Ms. K-9 America." Yes, a haughty appearing standard poodle was decked out with an ermine (hopefully fake) fur neckpiece and a diamond (certainly fake) studded crown. This aroused smiles from both my parents, which was no mean task for my depression-plagued mom. You could sense her smile but her lips never parted.

The final "entrant" was a rottweiler in a total body suit of black and white. My first reaction was to ask, "Why is your rottie dressed up as a dalmatian?"

The owner carefully turned her rottweiler to offer a side view which exposed a huge udder, and I immediately realized the "dalmatian" was a actually a "holstein cow."

At my request the proud owner walked around the bed to my mother's rocking chair. As soon as Mom saw what we had seen, her little smile turned into a teeth-exposing laugh, as she too noted those large breasts.

Being a large (if you know what I mean) Russian woman, Mom truly enjoyed the costume. It was a most memorable experience — one that I'll never forget. My mom died the following spring.

I first met Anne about twenty years ago and have been the
doctor for her canines all these years. Anne lost her second husband in 1998, and he too was a person I looked forward to seeing, partly because of his attitude with "Herman," their robust
seventy-five pound mixed shepherd.

"Doc, he doesn't like it here, will bite, and I can handle him
but give me a muzzle," he'd remind me during each visit.

I love clients who are not embarrassed just because their
pets don't like a veterinary office and may be aggressive about
it. Sounds like me in the dentist's chair — but no muzzle
required!

Recently, Anne, who is a retired schoolteacher, was hired to
do restaurant reviews for a classy local publication — *Lehigh
Valley Magazine*. As she related her new career status to me, I
mentioned that I had taken a few cooking classes myself.

Our vet tech, Julie, and I had attended four Italian culinary
classes as a diversion. (She probably could have taught the
course but was a good sport to accompany me.) Julie knew Anne
well as she had been a longtime client. On one of Anne's visits,
I mentioned that my meatballs were "pretty darn good" accord-
ing to my wife and daughters.

When the next issue of the magazine appeared, Anne, coincidentally, came in with a new bichon friese pup. The usual hug
and puppy fussing opened her twenty-minute visit.

"Well, did you read my most recent review?" she asked.

When it was apparent that I hadn't, she added, "When you
get the opportunity, be sure to read it. The last paragraph might
surprise you."

When that last paragraph started with "I took my dog to. . ."
I knew this was trouble. It ended with a recommendation for me
not to quit my day job but not before it alluded to my "wicked
meatballs."

The following Saturday afternoon after several hours dutifully spent in the kitchen, I delivered to said food critic my meatballs and marinara sauce made totally from the basil, garlic, and Italian parsley out of our garden.

In her beautiful thank-you note Anne shared the perspective that she lived by: "Cook only for family and for non-critical good friends — which are few and far between." Her advice has always stayed with me and has continued to motivate my joyful kitchen exploits.

When our daughters were six years old, they spent a few days with my parents. After we retrieved them, they greeted us with, "Did you know that Nanny and Pop Pop had to get married?"

Believe you me, at the first opportunity we called my mother and asked her if she realized what she had told her granddaughters. I had been raised to believe that way back then it was a sin even to *think* about doing *it* before marriage. My mother had said, "We rarely kissed except goodbye because one or both of my parents sat with us at all times." So where did our daughters get this scandalous idea?

The misconception started to come clear as my mother admitted to telling the girls that marriage was the only option for them to be together alone in the early 1930s. In actuality, she hadn't lied. As it turned out, she explained that she and her four sisters shared the same bedroom, and when her mom (my grandmother) had become pregnant again, there would be no room left for a new baby. So since she was dating my dad at the time, well, she simply *had* to marry him.

I love the process of recycling. There is something very grat-ifying about minimizing waste and maximizing care for the environment. Recycling can help some people in need and I like that too.

Today, our aggressive local community recycling program provides bins for just about anything and everything: telephone books, newsprint, cardboard, shiny paper, office paper, alu-minum, plastics, bottles, metal, and clothing. All this decreases punishment to our landfills.

My commitment to recycling goes back many years, before it was the socially acceptable thing to do. Mankind and Mother Nature provide wondrous proof of all that can be done when we understand the possibilities.

I'd never imagined that my involvement in recycling would ultimately focus on our house built in 1840. We decided to move when the neighboring cornfields were lost to high-density development, and the highway fronting our property was to be widened. Our strategy for meeting "progress" head on was to move house and home quite literally. If we would have left our house behind, it was doomed to be demolished and the site turned into a restaurant parking lot.

So to save this great structure and to avoid packing twenty-seven years of accumulations, we decided to relocate our 282-ton farmhouse to a new location. The move was a little more than a half mile across some cornfields to the first developed homesite in a charming subdivision where later new homes sprang up around us.

Our own house pets did us proud in 1993 during the move. Our three Burmese cats and one Lab were uprooted for three and a half months as we all moved in with a dear friend who welcomed us with open arms.

Moving a stone farmhouse is quite an undertaking. As my wife would eventually say, "We're thrilled that we did it, but once was enough."

Back in the days before the adjacent properties became macadam parking lots for town houses, we were surrounded by cornfields. Annually, in late November after the farmer would harvest his field corn, our Labradors would seek out kernels that had fallen to the ground from under the heavy farm machinery.

After Mother Nature would deliver her wintry blasts, Dinah and Bess would paw through the ice-encrusted field to get at the yellowed corn. Two days later from the rear windows of our farmhouse, we could see handsome pheasants pecking through our dog's bowel movements in search of the undigested treasures.

This was truly the ultimate in God's natural recycling program. The birds in no way could have effectively managed through the winter without a "warm meal" when they saw (or smelled) it. Another example of Mother Nature at her best.

When you are unable to breathe through your nose you tire easily and cannot taste anything. When this happens to a pet, he will find it difficult to accept oral medication. To overcome this, especially in cats, use Vicks VapoRub or Mentholatum in the nostrils. It certainly works for us to improve air flow though our noses.

Fifty years ago, if my brother or I had a sore throat, a stuffed-up nose, and felt sick, our mother would put BenGay on our necks and cover the area with a wrapped up T-shirt held in place by a safety pin. Sure it kept us warm but more importantly, it helped assure better air passage through our nostrils.

Now let's step back one more generation, long before these medications were available. This is how our mother described what her parents did for her and her four sisters.

My grandfather supported his family in the anthracite coal region of northeastern Pennsylvania by selling chickens and ducks that he had purchased live and then sold ready for the stove. I spent hours with him in his "poultry processing" enterprise.

When her daughters had a head cold, my grandmother would take fresh goose droppings, place them in a warmed towel, and wrap it around their throats. Guess what it accomplished? Clear nasal passages and a very quick recovery. (Did the five sisters just feign a cure to escape the dreaded treatment? I'll never know!) Ah, the healing power of natural remedies and another example of the benefits of recycling.

Periodically, calls come to our practice concerning the presence of ground hogs on someone's property that are uprooting a shed or decimating a vegetable garden. Whether digging or eating indiscriminately, they are a serious annoyance and need to be removed.

Conservationists know that these sylvan residents are extremely fastidious about their personal hygiene, so much so that people who study them have seen in their tunnels and underground dens separate chambers for their biologic wastes.

On the basis of this information, I have helped a few clients over the years with a proven technique to discourage groundhog residency. I offer to give to my charges what I call "Doc's Ding Dong Dung," a forty-eight hour supply of the contents of the intestinal tract from one of our Labs.

This solid, all natural waste product would be placed in a plastic bag, then a brown paper bag, then a cardboard box, and then into the trunk of my car with written instructions to place (actually, dump) the contents into the nearest "illegally dug" groundhog hole. This forces the occupants to seek new quarters, hopefully in another region, well out of the neighborhood.

For twenty-six years we had a satellite clinic on the lower level of our barn built in the 1860s. It encompassed 600 square feet or one-third of the available space at ground level. The beams and stone walls were exposed adding to its charm, and it served as an effective "feeder" office for our main hospital facility. As time passed and the practice grew, larger facilities were needed.

On the day after our full-service hospital opened, one mile north of the satellite clinic, we started the process of recycling our barn. A professional restorer of some note began the careful, precision process of dismantling the wonderful structure.

The art of taking this historic barn apart, piece by piece, was a community attraction, causing passersby to stop and watch the project in progress. The work of this small group of professionals caused your mind to wander a century back when skillful farmers labored to build for function and personal pride without the benefits of modern heavy equipment.

We were grateful that the barn was quite literally recycled into a stunning home one hour east of us in New Jersey — the home of people who loved and respected its connection with history.

This project in some small measure alleviated the sadness that each of our daughters expressed: "The barn helped raise us."

"Well now the barn is being raised — not razed," we replied. "Besides that, the office in it helped pay your college bills." Hence the beauty of the balance between structure and function.

Everyone has a story. Sometimes it takes the passage of many years for our respective stories to take shape and make sense. Regardless of who we are or what we've done, we are the product of a biological family and the eventual contributor to a family of our own making — whether by blood or affiliation. Whatever the case, a sense of belonging is vital to our happiness and connection in the world. Sometimes in the hectic pace of the world today and amid the challenges of relationships at all levels, our sense of belonging can be shaken.

No matter what our circumstances, pets are there for us, every day, no matter what. The bedrock of their unconditional love helps us to move forward to do what we need to do to build our lives. Our pets can give us great joy, can cause us worry, can bring us sorrow, and can make us laugh. At the very least they become and remain part of our life's story, no matter what — family members that never squabble or complain, who often help break the ice or ease the tension, who help us keep things in perspective, and who can keep us warm at night. Making pets part of our life story can help us create a happy ending.

EPILOGUE

If I Were the Vatican Veterinarian, the Official Dog Would Be the Labrador!

I confessed to you early on that the Labrador retriever is my favorite breed and by now you also know that I'm a practical man inclined to see the humorous twists and unusual connections in daily life. Am I guilty of a bit of hyperbole? Sometimes. Does that wee bit of exaggeration help us see things in a new and perhaps insightful way? I hope so.

As I consider my lifetime of caring for a gamut of pets, I have come to reflect on things from a philosophical, spiritual and applied point of view. I muse about my beloved Labrador breed and the great works to their credit — companion animals for the lonely or the visually impaired, partners in rescue work, and sniffers of contraband. I celebrate them for what's in their hearts: they live to give, to love and enliven, to comfort and forgive.

That said, I suspect it will come as no surprise to you that my fantasy job is to be the veterinarian for the Vatican where I would convince the authorities that the Labrador retriever should become their official breed — the ultimate canine representative of unconditional love. In order to win that prestigious designation, my arguments to authorities would need to be insightful, sensitive, and thorough. My evidence and logic would need to be impeccable and my knowledge of other breed candidates exhaustive. But I believe I am up to the challenge.

My strategy is to examine the key breed contenders, eliminating each one systematically. For starters I present two obvious choices — the Italian greyhound for its geographic connection and the Saint Bernard for its spiritual one.

Because of the location of the Vatican, both patriots and politicians alike would be appeased with the nomination of a "hometown boy," the Italian greyhound. The sprightly and spirited greyhound abounds in energy and is classically styled in the Italian tradition of elegant sculpting. These little guys maintain a refined attitude because of their long, graceful necks. Historically, they were found mummified in Egyptian tombs — certainly some religious mysteries are to be found in that fact. But wouldn't the size of this diminutive ball of fire be a liability in the cavernous Vatican? Wouldn't the dog all but disappear under the priestly robes of the cardinals as they sat and pondered the day's issues? Hence, I submit that this local boy has no place in the running.

Could there be any greater canine title for the official Vatican dog than "Saint," specifically the Saint Bernard? This hulking bruiser certainly could not find seclusion beneath the robes of Vatican residents. However, would the infamous, thick, slimy, salivary secretions be appreciated on their black outerwear? How would it look on the hanging tapestries? Or on the suit of a kneeling dignitary?

What veterinarian has not witnessed the walls of his exam room being covered with phlegm. And it always happens when wearing the navy blue slacks, not the khakis. Most Saint Bernards have ticklish, sensitive ears that produce head-shaking; that in turn releases those slimy missiles that are propelled over everything in their path. But is that risk worth taking to make the Saint the official Vatican canine? I suggest it is a legitimate nullifier.

Fortunately, there are other potential national favorites, many of which are lesser known but have important political and historical significance. The Italian hound reached Italy through the efforts of Phoenician naval forces. They became popular hunting dogs during the Renaissance. However, I just can't fathom the Vatican huntsmen in flowing robes mounted to the call of the hunt with the Italian hound poised to track or recover their prey.

Coming to Italy as early as the 13th century, the Bolognese was a very popular court dog. The word "court" refers not to the judicial system with those required stately robes but to court-*yards*. In these settings, this white cottony-coated, squarely-built breed is a wonderful companion dog, especially with children.

Because the church family at the Vatican does not include children, however, the Bolognese, being child deprived, would likely become depressed and require counseling — plenty of that available there. But courtly introductions could become challenging:

"May I present Baron Baldini from Bologna with his Bolognese Bridgetta." This Bichon-like breed just won't do.

For the Vatican some might suggest the mule-like Italian pointer known for its agility and hunting aptitude. The breed was so popular during the Renaissance that Italy often gave them as gifts to royalty and friends in France or Spain. Unlike the dreaded fruitcake gift, these dogs actually were highly desirable in spite of their stubborn nature. Perseverance would be an acceptable canine trait in this case, but not stubbornness. So I must rule out any breed with that quality.

Now the Spinone has a nice Italian ring to it. The breed is very much appreciated in Italy because it is multitalented, easily trained, and soft-mouthed. It appears on a 15th century fresco at the Ducal Palace in Mantua that depicts an early representative of the breed.

"Please pass the spumoni." "Another glass of Asti Spumante, perhaps?" No, the Spinone would be too easily misunderstood and confused within the fine eating and drinking tradition in the Vatican.

Let us consider the Neopolitan mastiff. In many respects it should be the front-runner for a place in the Vatican — calm, friendly, placid, stately. It's an ancient breed, dating back to the time of the Romans and the ultimate loyal guardian. It possesses a bear-like gait and a massive head. In addition, its prominent dewlap gives it the appearance of being multi-chinned. So herein lies the problem. Generally speaking, dog owners tend to take on the appearance of their canine companions. No stately leader of any sort would want to develop an enormous head or several chins, thus mirroring their dog. With such a hulking, massive companion dog, Omar the Tent Maker would have to become the Vatican tailor.

Since we have exhausted the local favorites, let's now consider another point of origin — Poland. This historically important nation played a key role in the geographical outcome of

Eastern Europe. It was a buffer state between Germany and Russia. So there are a few choices here.

The Polish lowland sheepdog has much the appearance of a bearded collie, is shy, and has an excellent memory. That's good and bad. He would have to have his beard in constant care to maintain a stately appearance — his own stylist perhaps. But it just wouldn't do. Imagine the Vatican barber declaring, "Our dog 'Stosh' is next in the chair."

All veterinarians know that lowland sheepdogs are a shy breed, sensing the personae of those around them. They have the innate ability to sense love, fear, kindness, and the like in people. Could it be some endorphin release? It would not look good if a demanding duchess visiting religious leaders had her shoes wetted by a submissive sheepdog. It would be unsuitable if it raised its hackles and bared its teeth as a resident priest knelt in prayer. This breed is a rule-out because of its remarkable sensing aptitude.

So what about the Tatra Mountain dog? This is a very large breed both in height and weight — a defensive-end type — and is surprisingly quick and agile. It was bred to withstand severe Polish winters and is a rugged representative of "caninedom." They have a placid nature but are prone to irritability. I'll help the authorities rule out this breed. The excellent Vatican heating system would be stifling to the Tatra and make for a very cranky dog.

Now, let us consider the Maresna sheepdog, also from Poland. The breed is both muscular and majestic with a bear-like head, and, as expected, is very powerful. Though not easy to train, the Maresna was descended from early flock guardians. The fact that Vatican religious leaders are *the* shepherds of their flocks allows this breed some brief consideration. But there is a problem. What global spiritual leader would want a poorly trained companion? This breed just won't do.

Mexico is a country offering important south of the border canine candidates for consideration and analysis. The Mexican hairless always takes a noble, stately stance indicative of the posture of those in leadership roles. But these dogs were utilized mainly as bed warmers. It would be a rather humbling experience if, during an audience with a prime minister, a servant interrupted and plucked José off the lap of a papal dignitary:

"So sorry, Father, your dog is needed to warm the minister's bed." This breed scores too low on the dignity scale.

How about the internationally-renowned Chihuahua? Though not of stately stature, this tiny breed epitomizes the small but powerful personality we see in many of our diminutive friends. What they lack in size they more than make up in attitude. Tough and tiny, they are classed as plucky. They can be sensitive to cold and shiver easily. Seemingly, they would enjoy the heat of the candles so typical of church services and the Vatican.

Bulletin: "The Vatican is saddened — not to mention embarrassed — by the disappearance of the Holy Chihuahua in the library's archives. The usual reward has been posted by the Burger's office." This dog's peewee size exposes it to the risk of getting lost or misplaced. And one must never rule out the potential for an international scandal caused by a canine kidnapping. Again, size is the deal breaker here.

That pretty much wraps up both the political and geographical choices for the premier Vatican canine post. Let's now give consideration to those dogs whose names in and of themselves might make them a strong option for selection.

The Pharaoh hound certainly must qualify. Egyptian by birthright, this representative of North Africa is regal in nature and tracks by both sight and sound; they even served as "guides for souls of the dead." Without adequate exercise they rapidly become overweight. Fat and immobile would be a poor image in service to the papal institution, to be sure. But they would be excellent partners for a priest's workout program.

The Cavalier King Charles spaniel's prestigious name itself lends well to the title of Official Vatican Pet. This breed is affectionate with very appealing large, dark eyes. But, just hold on a second here. There is no way I could support an Anglican breed. Scratch that entry.

The bloodhound is related to the Saint Hubert's hound and is another candidate for our study. Known for its friendliness, it just cannot wait to be with people. "Perfect," you might say. "As you wait for a priestly audience, you will likely be licked and salivated upon by the royal bloodhound." Because this breed is countenanced by a mournful expression, there is a risk that it might fail to uplift certain distressed visitors — a second reason for considering it an undesirable choice.

Being from Israel, the Canaan dog has a symbolic name that aligns it with a religious heritage. Its roots are based in the Middle East where it protected the tribal goats from jackals and other predators. The Canaan seems a suitable choice for the Vatican pup at first glance. But the curled-forward, undignified tail exposes its rear unfashionably. I can't imagine congratulating a papal leader on this selection. Would the call-name of "Levi" or "Jerome," so appropriate for an Israeli dog, sound right in Rome?

I must say, "No," to this candidate as well.

Let's next consider a breed purely on the basis of its name — the Great Dane. Developed in Germany, it is believed to have inherited its grace and agility from outcrossings with greyhounds. Enormous strength and size are combined with dignity and elegance. The long, chiseled face blends with a distinctive, intelligent expression. The breed is known for its affectionate nature and is very clean and easily groomed. They do, though, need space and a lot of food.

The first factor in rejecting the Dane would be its dietary volume and the associated expense. The high cost to maintain a giant breed's diet could be perceived negatively. Any parish priest would not look good saying, "Let's open wide our wallets and pocketbooks for the Vatican's 195-pound Great Dane, oops, I mean for the hungry in Central America."

The huge size of this class of dog means its longevity is short compared to the smaller breeds. Indeed, their life expectancy is only half as long as the toys. The "turnover" factor of the Great Dane puts it out of the running here also.

Now for my predictable pick — the Labrador retriever.

Their trainability is well documented by their accomplishments. They have served society well as guide dogs for both the sight- and hearing-impaired, drug and explosive detection, and search and rescue work following catastrophes. They also perform well as hunting partners and in competitions. They have few close seconds to their skills as therapy dogs.

Anatomically, the tail of the Labrador retriever is its most distinctive feature with a large diameter at the base and tapering all the way to a narrow tip; the wide nose and broad skull blend into a powerful neck. The tail should never be carried over the back nor should it have a curl in it. It should, however, be exactly coffee table height, always positioned to dust one clean, although servants abound at the Vatican, I'm told. Their expression is alert and intelligent and conveys a kind, friendly temperament. The Labs' most outstanding feature is that they are loving, people-oriented dogs. They are happiest when they are with you. They tend to be quite patient with children and wonderful family dogs. And just where is *the* "household" of a notably worldwide family? The Vatican.

I now put myself in a compromising situation. Labs are not particularly intelligent — trainable, yes, but intelligent, no. In fact, Labs rate low on the canine "S.A.T" test, compared to the big triumvirate of canine intelligentsia: 1, poodles, 2, German shepherds, and 3, Doberman pinschers. The good news is that the Labs' major attitude advantage is that they quickly grasp what you like and want them to do. Then they will try to please you to death. If you ever find a person like that, keep them as a friend or marry them, as appropriate!

Labs also make poor guard dogs. Fortunately, the Vatican is protected by well-trained, security people who just by their image command the respect of law-abiding people. So, the Vatican is securely positioned to invite in all who knock! They don't need canine coverage there.

In my fantasy attempts to convince the Vatican to declare the Labrador as their official dog, I imagine idealistically that the authorities would select not one, but three papal pups — a black, a yellow, and a chocolate Labrador.

"Let's see, we have a funeral service today, so groom well the regal black retriever; the calendar shows that tomorrow starts the celebration of Easter, therefore, prepare the yellow Lab for this the season of white. I also see that the day after tomorrow our Boy Scout Explorer Post will be here in full uniform — make ready the chocolate."

In my fantasy job and in my real life profession as a veterinarian, my wish for all religious and political leaders worldwide and for every person, you in particular, is the opportunity to give and receive unconditional love. Yes, my wish is for all people to discover what it means to receive more than they give through that special relationship with companion animals.

I have shared with you the gifts of love that I have received from our Labs and our cats, but you will hear the echoes of my stories from people who have entered into their own love relationships with every breed. Just remember, you have your own gift of love to share and others need to share their love with you. This has been my love story. It's a story without end. I hope it will remind you of the love story that is in your life today and one that will sustain you for all your days.

A FINAL TRIBUTE

She Never Stopped Giving.

Over forty some years, we enjoyed the love and companionship of six Labrador retrievers. But one of them remains first in my thoughts and in my heart. Her name is "Jemima."

Throughout my years in practice I have shared many sorrowful moments with wonderful clients who have had to say goodbye to their best of animal friends. On those occasions I share my story about Jemima. Here are the words I wrote in 1981 on the day she died and before my own tears had dried. It is my memorial tribute to how *She Never Stopped Giving.*

It was September 1967 when we moved into an old farm house where we still live today. One of my most prized possessions to accompany me in that move was Jemima, a cuddly, lively, curious black Labrador who was a mere eleven weeks old.

At that early age she was already giving us a boundless love that we had never before known in a dog, companionship beyond compare, and a mutual respect for each other's needs. (She also gave us fits when she dug in the yard and wandered off into the surrounding cornfields. True, she wasn't perfect — but close.)

As life began to fall into a more normal routine in our household, our twins, Alissa and Debbie, were born to us near Thanksgiving Day, 1969. Predictably, we used nearly seven years of "doggie talk" to calm our two new babies, so we shouldn't have been surprised when Jemima would hear our chatter and push her way into our laps, nestling between two screaming infants. "Hey, what did you expect? I always respond to cuddly talk," she groaned.

Jemima helped us raise our daughters with kindness and love as you might expect from a Lab. She was such a giving dog — a wag of her tail to knock down a fifteen-month-old new to the art of standing or that fuzzy tail in the face of a crawler. Yes, she was a giver, not a taker — except when lying beneath those high chairs at mealtime. She also gave us countless ground hogs proudly presented near the back porch. Jemima demonstrated a great deal of pride during her middle years.

She then gave love and attention to "Dinah," our third Lab, and helped train her. Later she endured Dinah's litter and our keeping of "Bess." She tolerated Bess beautifully and ultimately became part of Bess — she was her pillow.

But sadly, all love stories reach an end. This morning my wife and daughters said goodbye to Jemima. I dug a grave in our garden and then knelt on the kitchen floor alone with my dog. As my tears dripped onto her face, I explained that when life becomes burdensome and painful beyond remedy, it is selfish of us to keep her alive for our own sakes. I only wished selfishly that she might have fallen asleep forever by herself.

As I placed a tourniquet on her leg, she raised her head toward me, slowly and with difficulty. For some odd reason, the syringe would not function and the overdose of euthanizing anesthesia would not release. I went back to the animal clinic for a new needle. Upon my return, I found Jemima had begun to die on her own. In those few minutes when I was not by her side, she had become totally nonresponsive. Her weak, erratic heart was barely palpable. She had no reflexes. I did an immediate venapuncture to administer the solution, and she instantly and peacefully died in my arms.

As she was in life, she was also in her death: she just would never stop giving. She made her end as painless for me as I tried to make it for her.

A big, old stuffed dog now stands guard graveside as I sit here crying. In two days it will be Thanksgiving and again I will count my blessings. One of them is and will always be Jemima.

In Memory of
"Jemima"
1967-1981